Eating Free Ha
More Than 2,000 Peo
and Keep It Off

"I can't really believe I am a weight loss success story. I have been trying to lose weight for 15 years. I have tried every diet imaginable, always on the quest to lose 15 to 20 pounds. I starved myself for years until I met Manuel. He has taught me how to eat. He has taught me how to live. He has given me the tools to a healthy new lifestyle that I love. I have gone from a size 12 to a size 4. I am in awe of what I have learned. Manuel truly changed by life."

Stephanie, age 40, lost 25 pounds

"What kind of results can you get with *Eating Free*? I have dropped 182 pounds. My confidence has returned. I am no longer taking pain medicine for my back. I am stronger physically and emotionally. And my relationship with food has changed. I've learned a better way of living. I could not have done it without Manuel and his *Eating Free* program. Thank you, Manuel, for giving me a new life."

Kevin, age 48, lost 182 pounds

"I have learned a way of eating that will stay with me for the rest of my life."

Samantha, age 26, lost 40 pounds

"I ran marathons, competed in triathlons, read other protein-based diet books, and just about everything else I could get my hands on. No matter what I did, I couldn't seem to drop any weight. Manuel was the first person to actually help me achieve my goals. It was relatively easy compared to what I had been doing. The online tracking was extremely useful, and the plan was customized for me and my unique needs."

Eric, age 32, lost 50 pounds

"I have been obese and trying to lose weight since I was a child. I finally started the *Eating Free* plan when I was 37 years old and 261 pounds. *Eating Free* helped me lose 60 pounds over the last 9 months! I've tried so many of the other programs out there, but this is the first one that made sense to me. Manuel taught me more than just portion sizes and food groups; he taught me how the body works. There's no magic here: Manuel just gives you the knowledge, tools, and support to get you to your goals."

Kelley, age 38, lost 60 pounds

"I have had a weight problem my entire life. I have lost weight in the past on some 'extreme' programs, but invariably when I would return to 'regular' eating the next peak always seemed higher than the last. When I walked into Manuel's office eleven months ago, on the advice of a good friend, I had reached a new high weight, had little energy, and was suffering from a variety of weight-related physical ailments, including a bad back. The program that Manuel developed for me has come to feel much less like a diet and more like a new way of life, certainly a new relationship with food. In 11 months I have lost almost 70 pounds and my waist is more than 10 inches smaller. (And I am now buying clothes at Nordstrom's instead of the Big & Tall places!) *Eating Free*'s supportive approach and gentle coaching has truly changed my life."

Arthur, age 54, lost 70 pounds

"As head of global operations for a major consulting firm, I never seemed to have time to focus on eating healthy and, as such, had been steadily gaining weight for years. My doctor told me it was time to make a change and so I contacted Manuel Villacorta. I have been working with Manuel now for 7 months and couldn't be happier with the results. I have lost 27 pounds, lost 6 inches in my waistline and my percentage body fat is down from over 26 to under 13%. In addition, my overall cholesterol is now in the normal range with my good cholesterol rising from 41 to 59 and my bad cholesterol falling from 151 to 129. The key to all of this was that Manuel provided me with the tools and knowledge required to make healthy choices."

Steven, age 43, lost 27 pounds

"I still can't believe and can't get used to the fact that I not only lost 38 pounds but how easy it was. I feel as though I am in my twenties again and haven't felt this great in years."

David, age 48, lost 38 pounds

"When my trainer told me that diet was 80 percent of my fitness program, I went to see Manuel. It was only when I followed his program I started to lose those pounds, and more importantly, my body fat percent dropped within a few weeks from 31 percent to 27 percent. With my new diet style and training, my cholesterol dropped 40 points in four months, something I couldn't do for years! Manuel teaches you to eat with common sense without losing the joy of eating."

Marilyn, age 46, lost 15 pounds

"I have done many diets before, but *Eating Free* has been a life-changer for me."

Lois, age 32, lost 13 pounds

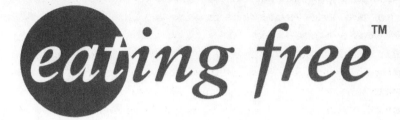

eating free™

The **Carb-Friendly** Approach to
Lose Inches,
Embrace Your Hunger, and
Keep the Weight Off for Good

Manuel Villacorta, RD, MS, CSSD

Health Communications, Inc.
Deerfield Beach, Florida

www.hcibooks.com

Library of Congress Cataloging-in-Publication Data

Villacorta, Manuel.
  Eating free : the carb-friendly approach to lose inches, embrace your hunger, and keep the weight off for good / Manuel Villacorta.
    p. cm.
  Includes bibliographical references.
  ISBN 978-0-7573-1635-7 (pbk.)
  ISBN 0-7573-1635-2 (pbk.)
  ISBN 978-0-7573-1636-4 (ebook)
  ISBN 0-7573-1636-0 (ebook)
  1. Reducing diets. 2. Weight loss. 3. Reducing diets--Recipes. I. Title.
  RM222.2.V497 2012
  613.2'5—dc23

                                                                    2012002220

Publisher: Health Communications, Inc.
        3201 S.W. 15th Street
        Deerfield Beach, FL 33442–8190

Cover photo ©Jun Belen
Cover design by Larissa Hise Henoch
Interior design and formatting by Lawna Patterson Oldfield

Contents

Acknowledgments

I AM EXTREMELY GRATEFUL TO ALL the MV Nutrition clients who have embraced my program. I've learned so much from their barriers, struggles, and successes. Their stories, pain, victories, emotions, laughter, and tears inspired me to create *Eating Free*. So many asked me when I would write this book. Finally, it's here and I dedicate this effort to the clients of MV Nutrition.

I am so glad to have met Jamie Shaw, who assisted me in writing *Eating Free*. She brought my research, science, and stories to life, and she is an amazing writer. Thank you, Jamie, for your hard work and persistence from book proposal to finished product. Thank you for believing in me and my message.

Many thanks to my literary agent, Andrea Hurst, for finding the perfect home for *Eating Free* at Health Communications, Inc. And to my supportive editor, Allison Janse, a great team player who honored my vision from the Eating Free message to the book design.

I'm also extremely thankful for my MV Nutrition team, the Eating Free family: Sarah Koszyk, RD; Sharon Kong, RD; Kelly Powers, intern, and Glenys Oyston, intern. This extraordinary and loyal team helped me with meal planning, recipe development, nutrient, analysis and constant support around "the book." Thank you to my friend Jun

Belen for the exceptional food styling and photography that made my dream cover a reality.

Finally, thank you to "mi familia" for their unwavering support. My mother, father, Erick, and Jeff. Without you, I would not be where I am. You gave me my strong foundation and the values of caring and giving. Your continuous love and support keeps me going, and I am who I am because of you.

Introduction:
My Journey to Eating Free

RIGHT NOW IN AMERICA, 47 percent of people are trying to lose weight, a statistic that actually seems low based on my own experience as a registered dietitian. The average woman spends thirty-two *years* of her life on a diet, while the average man spends approximately twenty-eight years trying to lose weight. But for all that time and effort, 64 percent of us gain the weight back. We try other diet plans, all based around eliminating different or additional foods. However, if I followed a plan based on what my clients tell me they've cut out of their own diets over the years, I would eat no potatoes, rice, pasta, bread, meats, chocolate, milk, fruit, bananas, carrots, corn, cheese, and more. The list of noes is, frankly, endless. All of these noes have killed the sacred tradition of eating and have elevated fear, guilt, and a negative relationship with our own self-image and the food we eat (or don't eat). The truth is, there's nothing wrong with eating any of these foods. Do we honestly believe that carrots, bananas, and potatoes are making us fat? Must we cut out bread and cheese altogether? Don't tell that to the French.

These sweeping generalizations are based on misinformation and a sort of cultural brainwashing from celebrity culture and the diet industry. Here's a big revelation: we don't need to cut out whole categories of foods and ingredients to lose weight. With Eating Free, you'll return to foods you love and celebrate eating again—all while losing one to three pounds a week, happily, healthily, and easily. I'm going to teach you how to integrate your favorite foods into a well-balanced plan that pairs foods in varied combinations with varied frequency.

Eating was hardly a concern for me, growing up in Peru. Preparing and eating a meal was as normal and necessary as, well, breathing! It never occurred to me to plan when or how to eat. I woke up, I ate breakfast, I got hungry, I ate lunch, and then, when I got hungry again, I had a snack. The day ended and I had dinner. Plain and simple.

Then, as a young man, I moved to America. The bustle of San Francisco was so exciting and new. Swept up in all things American, I found the social dining behaviors extremely fascinating. Eating was not an unconscious act here—it was a practice fraught with rules that people obsessed about. Suddenly, there were all sorts of foods I was told to avoid, including meat, rice, potatoes, bread, sweets, chocolate, and sometimes even fruit—all the staples of my native childhood diet. I learned that, for discipline's sake, I wasn't supposed to eat when I was hungry. Snacking was taboo. And since I was so busy with school, eating became the last priority on my to-do list.

At the time, gym culture was the rage. Forget spending time outdoors. It was all about the treadmill, weights, protein bars, and powders. And guess who started packing on the pounds? In fact, I gained fifteen pounds in my first year here. Isn't it interesting that once I began to obsess about weight, I actually started gaining?

Convenience stores, sandwich shops, cafés, and restaurants were abundant. Since I didn't know how to cook, I ate out regularly. No longer was going out to eat a celebration; it became a commonplace activity. In my youth, I sat down to eat with the family at *almuerzo*, our regularly scheduled lunchtime, which was more like a grand dinner feast. Everyone stopped what they were doing to come home and eat a hot meal together. Yet here I was in this new "land of opportunity," standing up, eating a prepackaged sandwich alone. How depressing! Despite my displeasure, I grabbed sandwiches and ate on the run—such a foreign concept considering how I'd been brought up.

No matter how hard I tried to acclimate, I hated eating a cold sandwich for lunch. I ate less, I slept less, I gained stress, and I gained more weight. I knew instinctively that something was wrong, so I wrote a letter to my mother (this was before the advent of e-mail) and asked her to send my favorite recipes from home. I knew I needed to learn to cook if I wanted to enjoy the quality of food—and the act of eating—as I had in my younger years.

• • • •

Since childhood, I've always wanted to help people. In the wake of my eye-opening American adventure, I entered the University of California, Berkeley, to complete an undergraduate degree in pre-med so I might follow a healing path. At the same time, I began using my mother's recipes that came in the mail, and I slowly taught myself to cook. It wasn't easy at first, but I figured out pretty quickly that I shouldn't cook meat on high settings unless I wanted dry, burned chicken. In any case, food became my primary interest as I was simultaneously learning all about the body. Quite organically, the two worlds collided. I came to understand that what we eat is at the root of form, function, and disease, the cause and the cure, and that my healing quest would come through food. It was my "aha" moment! It's when I knew my medical path would turn toward dietetics.

In the last six years of private practice, and the ten years prior, which I spent in public health nutrition work, I've learned an enormous amount of information. I have not only witnessed a physiological manifestation of a fat, starving nation but also the strength of the human spirit to endure extreme exhaustion. Time and again, my clients tell me what they don't eat, what they've cut out, how long they spend at the gym, and how well they can survive on next to nothing. Astonishingly, the glorious, pleasurable food that nourishes us is now tainted by guilt and fear. I am deeply saddened and disturbed by this modern trend, which people wear like a badge of honor.

I recently worked with an American couple who moved to Italy and found that they lost weight, even though they'd introduced more pasta into their diet and eaten it quite frequently. Upon returning to the United States, they regained their weight and more. This is a situation I've seen repeatedly, and I attribute it to a number of factors, from smaller portion sizes to a more relaxed pace of eating. While living abroad, they had adopted the native eating behaviors and actually found a healthier relationship with food. When they came home, they slid back into old habits and increased portion sizes, ate on the go, and used poor substitutions for whole foods. It was easy for me to see what had happened, but because of the prevalent myths we hear so frequently, this couple only focused on the fact that they'd eaten pasta while overseas, which was a very reductive perspective and one that had little to do with the reality of their weight gain.

Additionally, the woman told me she didn't understand why she'd gained weight upon returning home since she often substituted meals with healthy juices fortified with superfoods from a chain store. She seemed surprised when I pointed out that she was probably consuming twenty-four-ounce juices with added yogurt, sherbet, and possibly added sweeteners as well. It sounds so straightforward, but it's amazing the things people overlook when they're convinced they're "eating healthy." I hear myself saying it over and over again: "Eating healthy isn't the same as eating for weight loss." And much of the time, things we classify as "healthy" simply aren't.

With Eating Free, we are going to bring back the tradition of eating with all its joy, meaning, and celebratory associations—and still lose between one to three pounds a week. Our modern lives are often hectic and mindless, jumping from work to family to social and community obligations. So it's important we take the time to nourish ourselves—body and spirit.

Many of us have lost touch with what food is and what it does. For many, it is merely a means to lessen hunger, rather than to nourish. Despite the modern technological, medical, and even social advancements of our time, many of us find ourselves enslaved by food.

There is not a single day that goes by that I am not affected by the fear, guilt, frustration, and confusion of my overworked, overstressed, and undernourished clients. With this book, I'm hoping to put an end to all that. If you're ready to be free of the grind, the hunger, the frustration, and the pain, this book is for you. If you're ready to embrace your quality of life through taste and flavor, rest and relaxation, and thoughtful and joyous eating, plus positive, mindful steps, I can help you lose weight, now and forever. Eating Free is not a diet, a fad, or a trend. It's a lifestyle—and one you are going to love!

PART ONE:

• • • • • • • • •

The Eating Free Philosophy

Food

Rest

Energy

Expenditure

Chapter 1

Why Everything You've Been Told about Weight Loss Is Wrong

AS I THOUGHT ABOUT WRITING THIS BOOK, I pondered how much our culture has misled us about weight loss in the last twenty years. I only need to share the story of Amanda, a forty-year-old lawyer who came to my private practice hoping to lose twenty-five pounds, to illustrate my point. Amanda arrived at my office knowledgeable about nutrition and healthy, wholesome eating. She had already calculated how many calories she needed to eat per day and how much she needed to burn with exercise to lose weight. She even arrived ready to go with a 1,400-calorie daily plan. It was her intention to eat mostly organic foods, many prepared by organic supermarkets, with a focus on fruits and vegetables, heart-healthy fats, and lean meats. Amanda really just wanted me to validate her program and coach her through it.

Together, we discussed her demanding job, which required her to work at least fifty hours per week including weekends. I was surprised to hear that in addition to long work hours, she also maintained a strict exercise regimen of six times per week in the mornings before work (two spinning classes, two circuit training sessions, and two runs, for a total of about six hours per week). She assured me that she knew she should eat breakfast every day, so on her way out of the gym, she'd grab a protein shake and a banana and eat them in the car on her way to work—a very time-efficient solution. All her work and fitness requirements meant she had to follow a tight schedule, so to fit it all into twenty-four hours, she went to bed at 11:00 PM and woke up at 5:30 AM.

While at work, she had lunch when she felt hungry and when she craved sugar, about five hours after her breakfast. As a rule, she ordered a salad with chicken breast and dressing on the side. And, of course, she avoided carbohydrates at all costs.

By 4:00 PM almost every afternoon, Amanda experienced intense sugar cravings and, instead, ate a handful of nuts. She told me she suffered from sugar addiction, but fought her pangs by relying on her strong will-power. She avoided her favorite foods, such as grilled cheese and pizza, completely. She knew these were poor diet choices, and she was happy to make the sacrifice in order to lose weight.

So, you may be asking yourself, what did Amanda need with me, a registered dietitian, when she came in so full of knowledge about how to lose weight? The truth is she needed me to set her straight. After three months of following her self-designed program and spending $2,500 on trainer and gym fees, she hadn't lost any weight. In fact, she had gained a pound. Her trainer told her not to worry because she was muscular and muscle weighs more than fat. However, Amanda never wanted to gain muscle; she wanted to lose fat.

After investing all this time and money, restricting her food choices, and killing herself with exercise, she actually gained weight. Feeling angry and sorry for herself, Amanda went on a sweets binge. Then she came to see me.

So what was the problem? Doesn't it seem unbelievable that Amanda could work so hard and sacrifice so much, all in vain? Wasn't she doing everything one person possibly could to shed pounds? Her problem was the same scenario I've seen time and time again in my private practice. Amanda had diligently created a weight-loss plan based on the best information available to her via common culture channels like popular diets, TV programs, celebrity secrets, and gym culture fads. Unfortunately, that information was wrong.

Amanda felt confident she understood how to shed extra pounds through tried and true methods that we've all been hearing about for years. (Limit calories! Avoid carbs! Work out five times a week! Quit snacking! Avoid the foods you love!) But the reality is that she hadn't a clue. Much of what seemed intuitive to her, based on what she'd always believed, was, in fact, her downfall. Like many of my clients, Amanda arrived at my practice fatigued, frustrated, hungry, and angry—so much work and so little to show for it.

After years of seeing the same story time and time again, I knew this country was in crisis. Not only are we sorely overweight as a nation, we are sorely misinformed. As much as it seems like Amanda knew what she was doing, science tells us otherwise. Weight loss is much more than just numbers and calories. Amanda's view of how to reach her goal was based solely on caloric intake and exercise. She had no idea that stress, sleep, time management, regular eating, and smart food choices play just as much of a role in weight loss as do calories. Amanda needed less exercise, more rest, and more frequent meals to jump-start her metabolism. She also needed a better balance of macronutrients from her food.

It wasn't her lack of understanding about caloric guidelines or her lack of willpower. She demonstrated enviable willpower in avoiding everything she loved. She also gave up sleep, relaxation, and mealtimes to exercise. And she gave up her happiness. She effectively created a calorie deficit, but with Amanda, like so many of my clients, that simply wasn't enough. She wasn't really eating. She stressed her body. She slammed down a banana and a lab-engineered shake. She ate in the car. And she wondered what she was doing wrong.

In my sixteen years of experience, I've seen countless instances in which clients neglect factors beyond caloric intake, and as a result they inhibit or even reverse weight loss. The lesson is clear: only through a balanced, holistic approach can you expect steady, sustainable weight loss.

As a registered dietitian, I come to weight loss with two simple ideas as my guide: (1) the body needs fuel to survive, and (2) eating is one of life's greatest pleasures. Today our country is saturated with misinformation by ratings-driven media and a celebrity crush culture. Our ideas about particular food groups and exercise requirements are, to one in my profession, shockingly uninformed. In today's hyped up, get-skinny culture, we spend so much time trying to look like tabloid celebrities that we are willing to hurt our bodies and make ourselves miserable in the process. It's ironic that our pursuit of happiness via weight loss often just pushes us to depression, guilt, and self-loathing. The truth is we can be our very best selves without suffering in the process.

> Most of the methods touted for weight loss in recent years are based on denial and personal hardship—something contrary to everything the science of nutrition tells us (and contrary to our very human nature).

Additionally, most of the methods touted for weight loss in recent years are based on denial and personal hardship—something contrary to everything the science of nutrition tells us (and contrary to our very human nature). We need to eat. We want to eat. We should eat. And yet, everything in our culture tells us eating is like a dirty secret, a guilty pleasure that tempts us day in and day out.

Just think about the recent weight loss advice we've all heard. Avoid carbs. Eat only red meat. Avoid anything white, like potatoes, rice, or pasta. Forget about fats. Say no to wheat, dairy, potatoes, rice, carrots, corn, and fruits that are too high in sugar. Is there anything left we can eat? Let me share one anecdote that illustrates just how extreme our collective disorder has become. At times, Amanda subsisted mostly on almonds. She had avoided carbs at all cost for three years. *Three whole years!* She found this especially difficult because she loved potatoes in particular. When I told her that on my program she would be *required* to eat carbs, even her beloved potatoes, she actually started crying. And then, over the next many months with me, she proceeded to lose thirty pounds.

It's not healthy physically or psychologically to deprive ourselves in extreme ways. That's why I am so excited to introduce the new movement of Eating Free to this starving, overweight nation. The time has come to get back to eating—for nutrition, health, weight loss, and yes, for self-care. The program is named Eating Free because it teaches you how to eat free of guilt, deprivation, hunger, bingeing, fads, boredom, and yo-yo dieting.

This book will show you, chapter by chapter, how and why Amanda's flawed understanding represents our misguided cultural perceptions, all of which are derived from erroneous advice from various sources. With *Eating Free*, I will expose the truth about proper weight loss from a nutritional standpoint.

In addition to clearing up common misconceptions about how to lose weight, I aim to do something else with *Eating Free*. I want to restore a love of food and encourage eating as a way to strengthen bonds, celebrate life, take time to reflect and share gratitude, and generally enhance our quality of life. This approach to eating isn't just sensible and effective; it's personal to me.

Chapter 2

Embrace Your Hunger to Lose Weight

NOW THAT I'VE told you that everything you've been hearing for the past few decades is misleading, let's look at the science behind my claims. Please don't be turned off by the word "science." I hope you're going to find this information very empowering. Much of what I have to say will dramatically change how you view nutrition and weight loss. In fact, the information I'm about to share has only recently—in the past ten years or so—been discovered and proven by the scientific community. This means that the bulk of what we *thought* we knew about weight loss— particularly as it pertains to exercise—is just not accurate. But before we go into that, let's start with the basic mechanism that regulates our weight: *hunger*.

We all know what hunger is. We feel it every day to some degree. Hunger is really an essential strategy for survival. If you think about our body's functions as they relate to survival, it helps to remember what our bodies needed when we were a far more primitive species. Hunger and stress served as our basic survival skills. When we got hungry, we needed to eat. If the hunger got strong enough, we'd do anything to feed ourselves, including killing wild animals. We had to do it to survive. Without hunger, we would never have had the incentive, ingenuity, and bravery to do what it took to kill a potentially deadly beast. Stress also helped us to survive. If that beast decided to turn on us, stress gave us the adrenalin and cortisol we needed for fight or flight. Without these two physiological triggers, we never would have survived in the wild. So even though we live in a modern world, and we've evolved from a time when we had to kill our own food, our bodies are still programmed to behave in the same instinctual way.

In our environment today, everything from media outlets, to fad diets, to our friends encourages us to *fight* hunger. Not eating is considered to be a sign of strength and willpower, but remember, hunger is a survival instinct. It's the most basic thing we are programmed to do, and yet we're expending massive amounts of energy trying to stifle it. At the simplest level of this program, I want people to understand that it's okay to be hungry. It's okay to feed your hunger. In fact, I encourage everyone to embrace their hunger! We're supposed to be hungry, because our bodies need fuel to perform. Once we start denying our hunger, we're disturbing our body's ability to function properly—and that includes our body's ability to lose weight. So the first rule of Eating Free is: Don't punish yourself for experiencing hunger. Feed your hunger and recognize that it's a vital function. That may sound simple, but it's going to be a groundbreaking revelation for anyone out there who's accustomed to skipping meals and starving on a regular basis. I'm here to tell you, cut it out!

Now, before we go any further, let's make an important distinction. Hunger is not the same as *appetite*. Appetite is the *desire* to eat. While hunger is a cue from your body, appetite is a cue from your brain. Another way to think about this is that appetite is a luxury and a choice—a modern concept that appeared once humans had the option of choosing when and what they wanted to eat. Can you imagine one of our ancient ancestors, who wouldn't eat unless he killed a wild boar, saying, "Hmm, I think I'm craving Chinese food tonight"? That didn't happen. The concept of choosing to eat something specific would have been unthinkable—unless, of course, that individual was lucky enough to kill a hare and a boar on the same day.

> Hunger is not the same as *appetite*. Appetite is the *desire* to eat. While hunger is a cue from your body, appetite is a cue from your brain.

The point is, we often confuse hunger and appetite, and it's important, when learning how to lose weight, to know the difference. We often lump both concepts under "hunger," telling ourselves we are "hungry for Chinese food" when in fact we have an appetite for it. Maybe we are bored, stressed-out, or sad, and eating makes us feel better. That's behavioral eating, which happens for emotional reasons unrelated to true, survival-based hunger.

In addition to recognizing the difference between hunger and appetite, we need to acknowledge that *stress affects hunger*. That's part of that fight-or-flight scenario we explored earlier. We may not have to outrun wild animals these days, but we still have the same degree of stress—probably even more. In the wild, an animal chase may have occurred every once in a while, but we spend our modern days stressed from dawn till dusk: getting the kids ready for school, racing to work, dashing to the gym, trying to manage massive amounts of e-mails and deadlines, working long hours while trying to please the boss. Believe it or not, this sort of stress is equivalent to running from a predator, but these days, we're not burning it off by running away. These days, we're *feeding* the stress with doughnuts at work, caramel lattés on breaks, or martinis after hours.

When we're at ease, we produce the right balance of essential neurotransmitters: dopamine (which keeps us alert) and serotonin (which relaxes us). The proper balance of these two critical components keeps us content, alert, and happy throughout the day. But when we're stressed, this delicate balance gets thrown out of whack and can start to build fat around our waistlines. Why? Because when we get stressed, our cortisol levels increase and bring sugar into circulation from our cells. It happens because our bodies receive stress signals and assume, for instance, that a wild boar is chasing us, so it begins to fuel our muscles with sugar so we can outrun the beast.

But today, since we are sedentary—stressing more about work deadlines than hunting animals—that sugar goes straight to the liver and gets stored as fat around the waistline. So now our cells are empty *and* hungry. In addition, this release of cortisol makes us crave fat (because fat decreases cortisol). Chronic stress increases cortisol levels, and cortisol acts as a potent signal to the brain to increase appetite and cravings for certain foods, especially carbohydrates and fats.

Cortisol also acts as a signal to our fat cells to hold on to as much fat as they can and release as little fat as possible, even in the face of our attempts to reduce calorie intake for weight loss. If that weren't already bad enough for our weight-loss efforts, cortisol also slows the body's metabolic rate by blocking the effects of many of our most important metabolic hormones, including insulin (so blood sugar levels suffer and carb cravings follow); serotonin (so we feel fatigued and depressed); growth hormone (so we lose muscle and gain fat); and the sex hormones testosterone and estrogen (so our sex drive falls and we rarely feel "in the mood" when we're stressed-out and awash in cortisol). So, in sum, when you're stressed, you crave fat. Just as when you skip carbs, you crave sugar. So while we all think we're "addicted" to certain no-no foods, it's often just the case that we need to regulate what and when we eat. When we do this, our cravings disappear.

To make matters worse, the release of cortisol also decreases dopamine and serotonin, so it becomes harder to stay in balance and keep stress in check. Cortisol messes with our mood balance, and at the same time, it increases carbohydrate cravings and fat cravings, which may lead us to eat more chocolate, for example, in order to stimulate the low dopamine and serotonin. Now we've created a *reward system*. So from this point on, you'll crave that reward whenever you're sad or stressed, or even when you're happy. Your body will tell you it's just the thing to address your stress and cravings, so now you've created an unhealthy cycle that just feeds on itself. And just think: this could all be avoided by eating regular meals at regular intervals. It's pretty amazing when you look at what we do to avoid eating. If only we understood that by eating sensibly, we could lose weight and avoid the whole yo-yo phenomenon that tortures us time and time again.

In the scientific community, we call actual hunger *physiological hunger* (or *homeostatic hunger*). That's when your stomach is growling, you can't concentrate, and you're irritable and cranky. Your body is essentially demanding that you eat, and it will send you uncomfortable pangs until you do. It's your body trying to ensure its own survival. We refer to your appetite as *emotional hunger* or *hedonic hunger* (appetite), which is when you have cravings and longings for food. This is your brain asking you to eat. So with that fundamental dichotomy in mind, let's return to Amanda from Chapter 1.

Most of us would assume that Amanda was doing everything she should to lose weight. Even at this point though, just by understanding the difference between true hunger and appetite, we know that she was denying her hunger. She bragged about her willpower and fought her hunger all in the name of losing weight. On the Eating Free plan, she learned to respect and respond to her hunger. By learning how to pro-actively feed her hunger, she stopped her hunger hormone from raging, which drove her to binge.

Your Powerful Hunger Hormone

Did you notice I mentioned the "hunger hormone"? Did you even know we have a hunger hormone? I'll be honest—I didn't until about ten years ago. This is a relatively new discovery and one that has changed everything we thought we knew about weight loss. You see, our bodies secrete a hormone called *ghrelin*, which controls our hunger and drives our appetite. If we do not understand, monitor, and control our ghrelin, we can forget about losing weight. The truth is we don't give our bodies nearly enough credit. We think we can summon our willpower and dominate our bodies, but in reality, our hormones are exceedingly powerful. This is why it makes sense to respect them and work with them rather than fighting our bodies' basic instincts. When we skip meals and starve ourselves, we are at war with our bodies. And yet, we expect our bodies to conform to our desires to lose weight just because we will them to do so. Trust me, years of research prove that we will lose every time. Once we accept that our bodies know what they're doing, and work with our natural functions, losing weight becomes

> Our bodies secrete a hormone called *ghrelin*, which controls our hunger and drives our appetite. If we do not understand, monitor, and control our ghrelin, we can forget about losing weight.

much easier. While there are twenty-four different hormones that affect the appetite, we're going to focus on the one that increases appetite on a short-term, day-to-day basis, which is ghrelin.

Here's what we know about ghrelin today. It's a hormone secreted in the stomach when we are hungry. It is also known to increase appetite, so while the body is asking for food (and we are often denying it), ghrelin strategically triggers appetite in the brain. Why? Because we've trained ourselves to ignore a rumbling tummy, but once our brains get into the act, with our powerful imaginations fueling our appetite, it's far harder to resist food. We're dreaming of bagels, cheeseburgers, ice cream, and pizza. Never underestimate the power of the appetite to tempt us. It's an incredibly formidable foe.

Here we are, hungry, stomach growling, headache setting in, and our mood deteriorating by the minute. Our ghrelin is working hard, simultaneously increasing our appetite since we choose to ignore our physical hunger. What else is the ghrelin doing at this stage? It's decreasing our metabolism and our ability to burn fat. This is happening because the body is receiving signals that it's not going to be fed. In response, it begins to slow its processes and hang on to whatever stores of energy and fuel it's already got. While we're starving and fighting the hunger we feel, and dreaming of cheeseburgers, we're cueing our bodies to hold on to fat and to stop metabolizing what we've already eaten. Surely, this defeats the purpose of starving ourselves in the first place! The harder we try to avoid eating, the more desperately we want food, and meanwhile, our bodies are hanging on to fat and shutting down processing functions. Think of all of the people on diets who congratulate themselves for their incredible willpower while they're actually telling their bodies to hang on to that extra weight, just as their brains are preparing for an epic binge sometime in the near future.

Now, what most people don't know is that by simply eating a small meal every few hours, ghrelin levels are decreased. Studies show that carbohydrates are the best option to lower ghrelin, with proteins coming in second. This is because when you're not eating carbs, your glucose levels decrease. The brain feeds on glucose, so without it you end up craving sugars. I can't tell you how many of my clients come to me complaining of being addicted to sugar. Amanda said she experienced intense sugar cravings in the afternoons. Remember how she avoided carbs at all costs? That's why she craved the sugar. Her brain was shutting down because it didn't have the carbs it needed. Glucose levels were falling, so she began to crave sugar. Once we eventually got her regulated and "eating free" with a meal plan that included carbs, guess who stopped craving sugar?

I like to think of ghrelin as a little gremlin: a monster that lives inside us all. It needs to be fed constantly, at a slow, steady pace. When we ignore it or starve it, the gremlin goes out of control and begins fighting back. While you may hold tough for a while, eventually you are powerless against it. Hello, late-night binge!

Ghrelin Spikes

Research tells us that eating every three hours is about the right interval to manage ghrelin, which controls both hunger and appetite.

Ghrelin spikes when we wait more than three hours between meals or skip them. Research tells us that eating every three hours is about the right interval to manage ghrelin, which controls both hunger and appetite. Within thirty minutes after a meal, ghrelin begins to rise steadily until the next meal. Studies have shown that a longer break between meals is associated with a more significant increase in ghrelin production. Studies have also demonstrated that there is less ghrelin produced in the average person between breakfast and lunch (a three- to four-hour break) than between lunch and dinner (typically six hours), so timing the space between meals is a critical modulator of ghrelin.

We also know that ghrelin responds according to the amount of carbohydrates and protein in the body. Interestingly, water does not affect ghrelin at all. The myth that drinking water will fill you up is false, according to our hunger hormone. So eat! My recommendation to control ghrelin is to eat breakfast, eat every three to four hours, and mix carbs and protein during your meals and snacks.

Ghrelin spikes when we lose weight. Why? Because remember, your body only cares about survival. It wants homeostasis, or the status quo. Your body thinks losing weight is dangerous, so as you start to lose, you need to be extra mindful of your ghrelin function. Your body will fight back if you don't approach weight loss in a steady, sensible way, working *with* your ghrelin instead of against it. This is a fundamental principle to understand: you have to eat regularly to lose weight.

Ghrelin Spikes after Exercise, Especially in Females

Pay attention, ladies! When you exercise, your ghrelin spikes in order to preserve fat for biological birthing purposes. We'll go into more detail about the role of exercise in weight loss in Chapter 10, but I can tell you, with weight loss, it's far more important to monitor your nutritional intake than it is to exercise. I advocate exercise for everyone for health reasons, but it is not the primary way you're going to lose weight. For women in particular, an overemphasis on exercise during your program can actually *hinder* your weight loss if you're not monitoring and controlling your ghrelin. That's how important this hunger hormone is in your overall effort. Just know that when you exercise, that gremlin is going to act out, so you'd better be prepared to feed the monster before and after the exercise session.

Ghrelin Spikes Due to Lack of Sleep

This is a new finding, and one that surprises many of my clients. We now understand that depriving ourselves of sleep can impede weight loss or even cause weight gain. Why? Because the little gremlin is acting out again. It turns out the gremlin likes a solid six to eight hours of sleep a night, and if he doesn't get it, he's going to let us know he's unhappy by causing hunger and appetite to increase. Studies demonstrate that reducing sleep to four to five hours a night compared to longer periods of sleep (six to eight hours) increases ghrelin. People who sleep fewer hours get hungrier.

Now we know that we not only have to keep the ghrelin gremlin fed on a regular basis, but he wants some quality sleep time, too. Better give it to him, or he's going to start messing with our weight loss again.

Ghrelin Spikes from Low-Calorie Meals

The more we eat per meal, the less the ghrelin spikes. That doesn't mean you should be eating as much as possible; it means there is a minimum amount of calories you should consume per meal. Restricting meals to 200 calories for women and 350 for men won't cut it. You need to eat a minimum amount to maintain a healthy metabolism. That amount changes for each person, and as you get deeper into the book and begin to use my free record-keeping tool (either online or on paper), you'll discover your personal prescription. In order to access the online record-keeping tools, just join the free program and set up your account at www.eatingfree.com.

The point I'm making is that many of us think that the fewer calories we eat, the better off we are. This is simply not true. While we do need to cut calories—or create a caloric deficit—to lose weight, it's important we don't go too low. There's a popular fad diet right now that recommends that women eat 500 calories a day while taking hormone injections. Clearly, the hormone injections are tricking the body in some fashion, but I can tell you that 500 calories a day is never okay under *any* circumstances! This is a dangerously low amount to be consuming, and it poses all kinds of serious health risks. My clients know when they begin the Eating Free program that I'll prescribe a certain caloric goal for the day, but I'll also give them a baseline they should not dip below. I create an "optimal deficit" for every individual, which determines the amount they'll aim to eat, even if it means eating more than they even want to. Why? Because they're feeding the ghrelin gremlin, so he won't rise up and wreak havoc on their weight-loss efforts.

Ghrelin Spikes When You Avoid Carbs

Avoiding carbs or eating them in deficient amounts increases ghrelin, which in turn increases hunger and appetite, so just imagine what all these low-carb and carb-free diets are doing to your hunger and "willpower." It's not just that your body *wants* carbs; it's that your body *needs* carbs. More specifically, your brain *needs* carbs. The brain is just like a muscle that needs fuel. We've always known that carbs fuel us with energy for working out. That's why athletes talk about "carb-loading" before a big event. Now research shows that the average brain needs 130 grams of carbs per day to function optimally.

Think about this in the context of our evolution again. It's true that we're never going to be as active as we were in agricultural societies or during the Industrial Revolution when many worked hard-labor jobs. So it seems logical that we wouldn't need as many carbs these days. We are more sedentary, so we require less energy, right? Not really. Even though we're not as active, we still require carbs because now we're using more brainpower. And brainpower, like muscle power, requires energy.

You might think, "Who cares if my brainpower is waning, I just want to lose weight!" But the fact is our brains work in concert with our body processes, so when one is faltering, the other cannot function properly and achieve its goal. With Eating Free, you'll eat the right amount of carbs that your brain and body need. You have to take stock of your brain's carb intake because without the right amount, your brain will raise your appetite and send cravings for sugar, and you will gain weight. So guess what? Here's a weight-loss news flash: Not only are you *allowed* to eat carbs when losing weight, you *have to* eat carbs to lose weight. You need carbs.

> Not only are you *allowed* to eat carbs when losing weight, you *have to* eat carbs to lose weight.

Welcome home, potato. We've missed you, pasta. As we get deeper into the book, you'll learn which foods count as carbs and which carbs you should be favoring for optimal weight loss.

Taming the Self-Proclaimed Sugar Addiction

Many of my clients believe that they have intense sugar addictions. Nine times out of ten, the reason is because they've been avoiding carbs like crazy. Food is rewarding. So the less you give your body what it needs, the more it compensates with rewards, which are experienced as heightened, intensified experiences. I instruct those who claim to be sugar addicts to eat carbs, like oatmeal, at breakfast, some sandwich bread at lunch, fruit for a snack, or sweet potatoes with dinner. Within two weeks, they report magically, miraculously being "cured" of their sugar cravings. Actually, their brains aren't sending those sugar signals anymore because they've satiated themselves with the proper amount of carbs. What people don't understand is the cumulative effect of the myriad factors that trigger ghrelin, which in turn triggers appetite.

Let's look at how these factors converge in real life. Remember that when we get stressed, we increase our hunger. That increases cortisol and decreases serotonin, which in turn increases appetite. When we top it off by working out like a maniac, which increases ghrelin yet again, we compound the problem. Then we deprive ourselves of sleep (read: more ghrelin and more appetite). And finally, many of us avoid carbs, which increases ghrelin—and appetite—once more. What we need to remember is that spiking ghrelin isn't just a one-off occurrence. It's a nasty cycle that builds on itself and gets exponentially higher, raising our appetites to an insatiable level that will eventually drive us to eat everything in sight. You can bet that after such a vicious cycle, most of us won't reach for a cookie. Most of us end up going for a double cheeseburger, a large order of fries, and an extra-large milkshake. And that 3,500-calorie meal easily derails a whole week of what we have been led to believe is perfect weight-loss behavior.

In fact, many of us inadvertently prime our bodies for a downfall. It seems our most common weight-loss strategies these days actually end up sabotaging any kind of sustainable success. It sounds depressing, I know, but you should feel empowered, because with this knowledge, you'll start eating free and start losing weight for good this time.

There's one more term we should review before I teach you how to control ghrelin, and that's the word *metabolism*. We all use this word often, and most of us understand generally that it's the process that keeps us working, like a mechanical engine. While your heart is pumping, your blood is circulating and your brain is working, and your metabolism is working away, providing the energy you need for these functions. We call this the resting metabolic rate. When we sleep, the body slows down to preserve that energy, but the metabolism still works, so it still needs calories. Your body at rest becomes energy efficient and attempts to store fat around your waistline. But we don't want to be energy efficient. We want to be rapidly burning weight.

So to maximize burning, Eating Free will teach you to eat throughout the day to keep the ghrelin production under control and the metabolism humming along at full speed. It's important to monitor ghrelin because high ghrelin lowers your metabolism, and if you're not eating, that's a double whopper. By feeding your ghrelin steadily all day, you'll keep your metabolism strong so it's burning as much as possible. With Eating Free, you're eating more, and thus, you're burning more, even while you're asleep.

The Core Principles of Controlling Hunger

Eat breakfast within an hour of waking. Be sure your breakfast is a blend of carbohydrates, fiber, and protein. In Chapter 4, we'll be looking at food combinations and proper portion sizes. It's the most important meal and it drives your entire day. It determines how much you're going to eat at 4:00 PM. It will control ghrelin and set you up for success. If you exercise in the morning, maybe have a pre-exercise snack, like half a banana or a string cheese. This will increase your metabolism, help with clear thinking, improve alertness and concentration, enhance memory, and improve cognitive abilities.

Do not skip meals. There is a lot of contradictory research right now about mealtimes. Some people say you should eat three meals a day, while others say you should eat five or six. For many people, three square meals don't work anymore. These days, many of us wake up at 5:00 AM and stay up until midnight. Plus, we work harder and expend more brainpower, which uses up fuel. You need to eat every three to four hours to control ghrelin, so depending on how many waking hours you have, you may have four meals or you may have six.

At every meal or snack, try to combine carbohydrates and proteins. Because your food intake works on weekly averages, rather than daily (a concept we'll discuss at length later), the ratios at each particular meal or snack time are less important than the mere fact of consuming protein and carbs together. This way, you get the optimal blend of nutritional elements to fight cravings, control hunger, gain energy, and stimulate fullness. Protein increases your metabolism while carbs lower ghrelin, help with brain function, and decrease cravings. So instead of just reaching for an apple, add a piece of turkey or low-fat cheese. The food-combining aspect of my program can be as simple as that.

It doesn't matter what time you stop eating. It is a myth that we shouldn't eat after a certain time in the evening. Just give yourself at least ninety minutes before you plan to go to sleep. You need that ninety minutes to digest so you can sleep comfortably. I like to think of this as **the 70/30 Rule**, which means you should eat 70 percent of your calories before dinnertime and 30 percent at dinner, whatever time that may be.

Stay hydrated. You've heard it a million times, but drinking water is essential for keeping energy up, aiding the metabolism, burning fat, and more. It's the fluid your body needs for life, and it's an instrumental part in your weight loss. Other fluids can be useful, but water is obviously the best choice as it is calorie free. Forget about

> **The 70/30 Rule:**
> You should eat 70 percent of your calories before dinnertime and 30 percent at dinner, whatever time that may be.

that whole eight cups a day thing. I want you to relax and remember to have a healthy amount of water whenever you think of it. Thirst can confuse your sense of hunger so make sure you stay hydrated.

To review what we've learned in this chapter and look ahead to where we're going, let's sum it up. Weight loss is not just about excess food. It's attributable to hunger, appetite, hormones, a stressful and sedentary lifestyle, emotional eating, misinformation or confusion, an overemphasis on exercise, and lack of sleep. It's also due to other factors—like eating out and eating foods that cause an inflammatory response in your body. So with so many factors at play—from ghrelin, to food combining, to exercise, confusion, and all the rest—how can we possibly synthesize all this information and apply it to weight loss? How can we put it together in a simple, easy-to-follow plan that helps us balance all these factors while still enjoying life and eating foods we like? I'll explain it all in the coming chapters so you can learn how to actually apply my philosophy as it pertains to eating, exercising, resting, and de-stressing. The remainder of this book is divided into three parts. Part 2 is about food, Part 3 is about REST (*R*enew, *E*nergize, *S*leep, *T*ime for You), Part 4 concerns energy expenditures and the tool you need to track all of these components and their related behaviors.

PART TWO:

• • • • • • • •

Food

Chapter 3

Food Is Not Evil: Enjoy What You Love and Lose the Weight

RECENTLY I MADE MY GRANDMOTHER'S recipe for rice pudding from scratch using whole food products. Made with white rice, milk, and sugar, this fabulous Peruvian dish always fills my home with an incredible, aromatic sweetness. I am overwhelmed and moved by the warmth of the stove, the flavors and familiar smells comingling with thoughts of my childhood, my grandmother, and a simpler time of home-cooked meals. And inevitably, I can never escape the feeling of loss that makes me wonder what happened to food and to our tradition of eating.

Just as I learned nearly twenty-two years ago, mindfully selecting, preparing, and eating whole foods should be as cherished as the air we breathe. When did the concepts of eating on the go or devouring plastic-wrapped or boxed meals in a car become appropriate methods of dining? How did eating in front of the TV or in the car become alternatives to the dinner table? Our modern lives are often so hectic and mindless; we jump from work, to family, to social and community obligations. It's imperative we take the time to nourish ourselves—body and spirit.

The idea of returning to the pleasure of eating is fundamental to everything I teach. As a society, we avoid food and make ourselves feel guilty when we indulge. It's amazing to think that we demonize the very thing that sustains us and gives us the fuel to function, but it's an increasingly widespread trend that's overtaken our collective consciousness. Just think about the most popular diets in recent years. Some of the most well-known, doctor-endorsed plans call for cutting carbs almost entirely, in some cases by eating a diet primarily of protein, regardless of the fat content. Some of these plans prohibit white starches, like potatoes, pasta, and rice, or even worse, some new trend diets are telling us to cut out grains completely—and yet whole civilizations have subsisted on those staple foods for millennia without becoming obese.

To me, as a registered dietitian—and one who adores eating for pleasure—these approaches are reductive, robotic, and sometimes really dangerous. Besides denying users the right blend of macronutrients, these plans deny the pleasure of eating a varied, exciting blend of foods we crave and enjoy. And in many instances these plans create a fear of food, trigger disordered eating, and cause guilt for loving food.

As I've mentioned, I grew up in Peru, a fact that holds a powerful influence over how I perceive many aspects of life, but particularly my relationship with food. Not only did I eat what I wanted when I wanted, but I held reverence for mealtimes. We didn't only eat to subsist; we ate to celebrate, to honor family, to show gratitude, and to live in the present moment. Sadly, it is an approach that is on the decline or forgotten in our modern world. It's a concept I call "eating with elegance."

Eating with Elegance

In my mind, eating should be an act that awakens all the senses. With even the slightest attention to the experience, eating is filled with moments of pure, primal pleasure, from the first smells wafting from the kitchen to the sound of chopping, the vibrant colors of fresh produce, to heavenly textures and flavorful taste. Some of the most enjoyable moments of my life are punctuated by my heightened awareness of a perfectly tender scallop, the sweet smell of cakes baking, and the crackle of roasted chicken skin and the juicy, moist meat within.

When I think about how many clients come to me with stories of living on lettuce, diet bars, or protein shakes, I feel sad for them. I understand how desperately they desire to lose weight, but in the process, they haven't allowed time to actually eat properly, and they have robbed themselves of any pleasure from one of life's greatest gifts. In fact, I have clients who describe feeling "at war" with food or being in "food jail." What a sad way to live.

Eating with elegance is not only about the sensory pleasures of food—which are, in themselves, tremendous—but it is also about the mindfulness and care we apply while eating. So much of our culture is rushed that we scarcely consider how sacred and special the act of eating can be. One example of this is the presentation and polish surrounding a meal we create. Although I get up early to go to the gym, work a full day in my office, and then tend to other work, like public relations and meetings, I always make time to observe my lunchtime ritual. Much to the bemusement of clients, I use a glass bowl and silverware at the office, and not just a junky old fork someone found in a desk drawer. I have a set of fine silverware from home and a folded linen napkin I keep in my work kitchen for everyday use. It may seem silly or pretentious to some, but it's my way of honoring the moment, a way to celebrate the act of eating.

> Eating with elegance is not only about the sensory pleasures of food—which are, in themselves, tremendous—but it is also about the mindfulness and care we apply while eating.

A final element to consider when thinking about eating with elegance is the time spent eating food. In other countries like Italy, France, and, yes, Peru, people take two hours on average for lunch. Here, we typically take five to ten minutes. I'm not asking you to change your life and take two hours, but do take twenty minutes. Sit down. Chew your food. Be present and recognize the act of eating instead of shoving food down your throat while rushing from one meeting to the next.

A recent study in France showed that even when locals ate at McDonald's, they took an average of twenty-two minutes to eat. In a United States McDonald's, our average was fourteen minutes. It takes about twenty minutes for your stomach to send the message to your brain that it is satisfied. If you eat too quickly, your body will let you keep eating, and as a result, you will ingest more than your body needs. Your brain needs that reward, and it needs to know your body received the necessary nutrients.

When you're eating too fast, or on the go, your body and your brain don't get the reward of eating, so you never feel satisfied. Later, you crave not only food but also the time it should take to enjoy your food. My philosophy is built around the idea of taking the time to enjoy everything we eat.

As we begin to apply the Eating Free principles, please always remember that food is not evil. Food is synonymous with pleasure. Not only should we embrace food, we should anticipate eating it with excitement; we should relish the experience with joy, and we should feel contentment after we indulge, feeling fortunate to have enjoyed the moment. The reason we tend to avoid our favorite foods and feel guilt after eating them is that we've linked them to bad behavior. We deny and deny ourselves until we finally crack, and then we go crazy, bingeing on "forbidden food" as if we've never eaten before.

Our minds go haywire in that moment of gratification, telling us we'd better scarf down as much as possible since we aren't otherwise allowed this temptation. We don't know how to enjoy our favorite foods in moderation, which would allow us to embrace the experience of eating them occasionally with no repercussions and no negative associations. I don't believe in cutting things out entirely. I do believe in learning what proper portion size is and also learning smart ways to recreate our favorite cravings with slightly healthier ingredients—and trust me, I've got some great ones to share.

With Eating Free, 84 percent of clients keep their weight off after a year of losing weight. Losing the weight isn't the hard part—maintaining the weight loss is the real challenge. However, most of us never learned how to lose weight while eating what we love. Sure, you can lose weight if you cut out everything you like or avoid whole food groups, but how long can you really sustain that level of denial? According to my research: not very long.

With Eating Free, you'll learn to eat what you love and adopt a greater, more holistic approach to self-care. Rather than going on a diet and cutting wine, cheeseburgers, desserts, and more, I recommend learning how to integrate those foods and manage your intake. I advocate creating policies around your food intake, an effort that will help you liberate yourself from the slavery of dieting. Rather than avoiding your favorite cookies, create a policy like, "I will enjoy that cookie only on Saturdays when I meet my friends for coffee." Simple techniques like this retrain your brain to monitor what you eat without avoiding or demonizing it. If you enjoy a caloric food one day, watch your choices the next few days.

It sounds elementary, but in our culture of punishing ourselves for enjoying decadent foods, we tend to think to ourselves, *Well, I blew it Friday night, so the whole weekend is shot,* thus giving us permission to keep on bingeing for forty-eight more hours and saying, "I will start on Monday," and Monday never comes. With my approach, you will learn to control food so it doesn't control you. I'm here to tell you to take charge of your eating choices, empower yourself, and feel good about your decisions. Why? Because food is not the problem.

Pasta, Bread, and Potatoes Are Not the Problem

The increase in convenience foods is really where we see our collective downfall. While the United States leads the pack for obesity rates, we're seeing a global weight problem all around the world.

As you can see in the graph, Italy increased very little: 2 percent in ten years. The two countries that have increased most dramatically other than the U.S. are China and Peru. In rural areas of those countries, people are still eating primarily white rice in China and potatoes in Peru, and they don't gain weight. It's in the urban centers, which are now bursting with fast-food chains, where people are seeing a dramatic shift in their collective weight gain.

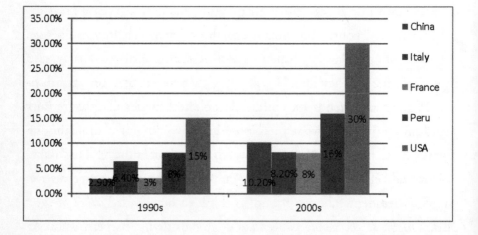

On first glance, we would probably assume that people are getting fatter in China due to rice, in France due to cheese, and in Italy due to pasta. But since these cultures have indulged in their signature foods for thousands of years, the idea that these ingredients are suddenly making people fat simply doesn't hold up. What *has* changed in these countries is access to fast food and greater influence from the American way of life, which rewards hard work, high stress, deprivation, and instant gratification. For example, due to Westernization, China is now making more money and eating more processed, fatty foods. We see that the biggest obesity problem happens in the metropolitan areas of these countries, like in Beijing.

However, people who have *some* knowledge of nutrition mistakenly assume that staples like fruits, rice, pasta, and potatoes raise your insulin and then make you fat. True, this may happen if you eat four cups of rice or eight cups of pasta. It *doesn't* happen if you eat a responsible portion. A normally functioning body is well able to process the right amount of carbs per meal. Carbs may also be a problem if you have prediabetes or insulin resistance and type 2 diabetes, but even then, if you know how much of a food you can eat, you can control those biological responses.

As you'll learn, the carbohydrate recommendation in Eating Free provides enough carbs to help people even with insulin resistance. I always recommend that everyone should eat as if they had diabetes or insulin resistance. Eating the right amounts of good carbs and protein throughout the day helps the body to not overproduce insulin and keeps your energy going. In my practice, hundreds have lost weight even though they had conditions like polycystic ovarian syndrome (PCOS), prediabetes, metabolic syndrome, and type 2 diabetes, which all had insulin resistance. To return to the international example, Italians eat pasta as their first meal, and they enjoy a very small amount by our standards. Then they eat a healthy portion of protein and veggies as the main course. Here, we eat pasta as our main meal—often a whole plateful—heaped with cheese and meatballs. The same is true of rice in Asia. It is meant to accompany a nice piece of meat and some vegetables, not be served as a main dish.

Where I grew up, every meal was served with potatoes and/or rice, two whole foods. In fact, in my native country, 70 percent of the calories consumed come from carbs like potatoes and rice. And yet, Peru didn't have many overweight citizens. When I tried to research the obesity statistics from those years, such studies didn't even exist. There simply wasn't an issue with weight gain across the populace. I clearly remember that in my graduating class of 1984, there were only two or three people out of 250 who were mildly overweight. No one was obese. Today, it's quite a different story.

In 1996, the first fast-food chains opened in Peru. On a recent visit, I made a note of the fast-food establishments I passed in a two-mile drive. In that short distance, I saw all the popular fast-food chains for burgers, pizza, doughnuts—you name it. It felt like I was driving on an American freeway. When I was growing up, there was one supermarket, and most people frequented the open markets or farmer's markets. Today, there are many modern supermarkets that carry processed junk, from sugared cereals, instant cake mixes, and instant noodle soups to highly processed snacks. I even saw one of my favorite Peruvian sauces (Huancaína sauce) in a "ready to eat" container, packaged with trans fats (hydrogenated oils). Does anyone wonder why Peru now has 16 percent obesity and 39 percent of the population is overweight? I can tell you—and it has nothing to do with potatoes, rice, bananas, yams, or milk.

I understand that you may be asking, "What does all this talk about Peru have to do with me?" The point is that looking at the traditional diets of faraway countries can tell us a lot about the health of a people, and seeing the rapid increase of obesity in a place that always subsisted on rice and potatoes demonstrates that those nutritious staples are not the problem. Processed foods in oversized portions are the problem.

Out-of-Control Portions

If you want to know what I consider to be ridiculously large portions, just turn on your TV. Restaurants strive to outdo one another with triple-decker sandwiches, half-pound burgers, pizza crusts stuffed with added cheese and meat, and more. We actually even have TV shows featuring restaurants around the country that serve the largest portions. It's all part of our consumer culture. "More" and "bigger" seems to equal "better" in so many spheres of our lives. One example that really crystallizes our excess is orange juice. I conducted a simple experiment, which confirmed all my beliefs about how far we've fallen in terms of knowing what and how much to eat.

While in Peru recently, I asked my mother for a glass of orange juice, and she proceeded to squeeze two fresh, sweet oranges into a five-ounce glass. The orange tasted ripe and flavorful, vibrant and satisfying. When I returned to the states, I visited a friend's home and asked him for some OJ. He pulled out a plastic gallon jug, got a sixteen-ounce glass, and filled it to the rim. He also set the jug down on the counter "for refills," just in case I wanted more. The idea that anyone needs that much juice with all its sugar is ludicrous. I love juice. Citrus is good for you. So have the juice, but don't serve yourself a massive portion. And if you have a choice, opt for fresh, real juice, if you can. You'll love the true flavor of the fruit versus the fake stuff loaded with extra sweeteners and preservatives.

Another example that illustrates our portion distortion is cake. Picture a normal-size nine-inch round carrot cake. In Europe, a cake that size is sliced to serve thirty people. In the United States, a cake that size might typically serve eight people. It's just another demonstration of how out of touch we are with what we need to feel satisfied and manage our weight. Just like the orange juice, I tell my clients to enjoy carrot cake, but first I teach them a proper portion size and explain how to plan a weekly schedule that accommodates occasional treats while staying on track to lose weight.

So what's the solution? Now that I've told you all the challenges we face in establishing a healthy relationship with food, we need to talk about solutions. I don't believe you should run from your favorite real foods. Rather, you should learn the right portion sizes and eat your chosen delights occasionally and mindfully. You may not be able to eat a five-inch slice of cake, and you may not be able to eat cake five days a week, but you also don't have to cut it out entirely as so many other weight-loss plans would have you believe. I'll always tell you to enjoy what you love and think about what you're eating. If you do, you'll feel rewarded and be more likely to stick with your program for the rest of the week instead of deciding you've blown it and throwing caution to the wind.

Eating What You Love Does Not Mean "All You Can Eat"

Eating what you love doesn't mean "all you can eat." Internalize that idea, and you're on your way to weight loss. My research shows that clients who ate one or two of their favorite forbidden foods a week still lost weight. Those who ate four or more pleasurable foods (meaning those higher in calories) plateaued or gained weight. Learning to incorporate what you love at the right frequencies will also help you understand how to moderate that

> Eating what you love doesn't mean "all you can eat."

food choice when you reach your goal weight. Remember that depriving yourself of food, especially what you love, makes you want it even more. Food is rewarding, and this reward feeling intensifies if you restrict.

Your Body Works on Weekly Averages

Your body works on weekly averages, so in any given week, one day will not kill your efforts toward weight loss. Many people have dessert one night and decide they've wrecked their diet, so they give themselves permission to binge and pick up again the following week. Instead, enjoy the treat, eat it with elegance, and then move on. Be proactive over the next few days to balance out what your body needs. You'll learn how to do this by understanding your weekly allotments and managing your entire week of eating. If more people just looked forward to the occasional dessert, enjoyed it without guilt, and moved on mindfully, they'd be able to snap right back into their weekly program.

Chapter 4

Newtrition: The Winning Combination Is 45-30-25

BECAUSE OF EVERYTHING WE'VE COVERED SO FAR—the relationship between hunger, appetite, ghrelin, and metabolism— science tells us we need to eat minimum amounts of each important food group for optimal brain and bodily function, as well as for weight loss. All the diets that tell you to avoid all fats and carbs are setting you up for physiological failure. I say, don't fight your biology. Give your body what it needs, and watch what you'll soon achieve. When it comes to eating right for weight loss, my research shows the optimal combination you need to fuel your brain and body—and achieve quality weight loss—is 45 percent carbs to 30 percent protein to 25 percent fats.

While it is possible to lose weight simply by imposing a caloric restriction, it may not be what I call *quality weight loss*. You may decrease muscle mass and bring on depression, hunger, cravings, and unsustainable behaviors. My 45–30–25 formula is designed to give you enough carbs to fuel your brain and prevent sugar cravings. It also delivers enough protein to prevent muscle breakdown, keep your metabolism going, and control ghrelin. Finally, it ensures you get the good fats you need for your health and that you enjoy what you eat.

As you begin to eat free, you will learn how to eat a balance of foods within your prescribed daily caloric amount. As you know, one of my philosophies is *eat more, not less*, and that will be accounted for in your personal plan. Within your caloric recommendation, you'll get food group allowances or "freebies" that will be allotted in the proper 45–30–25 amounts and portion sizes based on your metabolism and physical activity level. This way, you can be confident you're eating the optimal blend of nutrition types in the right amounts for quality, sustainable weight loss.

> When it comes to eating right for weight loss, the optimal combination you need to fuel your brain and body—and achieve quality weight loss— is 45 percent carbs to 30 percent protein to 25 percent fats.

The Eating Free plan is not only about calorie counting—it's about understanding what foods to eat and in what portions. Yes, you can lose weight simply by counting calories, but with a poor blend of nutritional groups, you could suffer mood swings, muscle loss, and uncontrollable cravings, all of which will derail or reverse your weight loss in the end. As you adopt the Eating Free program, you'll be learning about food—not calories. You'll identify what you like and learn how, when, and in what portions to eat it within weekly increments. If you follow the recommended amounts and distributions, you'll enjoy quality, lasting weight loss. This is what it means to be eating free. You're going to embrace your hunger, not stifle it.

Find Your Optimal Deficit

In order to create your custom plan, you'll start by finding your optimal deficit, which is a caloric restriction. It is a reality of weight loss that you need to cut calories for success. You've got to eat less than you're burning, period. But just cutting calories is not the answer, and this is not a calorie-counting plan. While you may be eating fewer calories than normal, you'll have plenty of fuel for the energy you need to sustain your day. I won't deprive you, make you feel hungry, or too greatly restrict the amount of calories so you later binge because you've been "good" (and miserable). You can find sample meal plans for certain types of people beginning on page 70. Or you can also get started today by calculating your own optimal deficit on my free website at www.eatingfree.com. Remember that you'll need to join the free program online to get your personalized prescription and your personalized optimal deficit. It's a simple four-step process to customize your plan and then you'll be on your way.

Eat What You Love

You're going to find that the 45–30–25 formula is the perfect blend of macronutrients to help your body function optimally for weight loss, while also making you feel full, satisfied, and energized—not deprived—because you're getting a wide variety of foods you love, not just what you consider to be diet foods. So whether you love burgers or pizza or burritos, you can have them; you just need to learn how to make them with smart ingredients in the right portions and how to balance them out throughout the week.

Looking at the chart below, you'll see a sample 1,600-calorie per day prescription, which is then broken down into freebies based on the 45–30–25 formula. This example also factors in an average of weekly exercise. You can use your freebies over the course of the week, aiming to spread them equally over the days, but sometimes eating more or less on specific dates depending on what you have planned. As long as the total adds up at the end of seven days, you'll be in good shape. This chart represents mere guidelines, and as long as you come within two percentage points (plus or minus) of your percentage goals, you'll continue to lose weight.

YOUR PLAN

Caloric Prescription	
Prescription	Calories per Day
Average From Food	1,600
Average From Exercise	300

Freebies	
Freebie	Quantity
Grains and Starches	5
Fruit	4
Milk	2
Non-Starchy Vegetables	5
Meat or Vegetarian Meat	11
Fat	6

Macronutrient Distribution	
Macronutrient	Quantity
Carbohydrates	45%
Protein	30%
Fat	25%

Learn Your Freebies

A freebie is the amount of food you are given to eat in a day, and because it's allotted, it's "free" for you to eat without guilt. So many typical dieters choose one or two "safe" foods, like lettuce and chicken, and that's all they eat. With Eating Free, you need to eat all the macronutrient food groups, not just for variety, but also because the combination of foods will help your body lose the weight. This also means you can eat a variety of foods you love. With Eating Free, you'll always know how many freebies you can eat within the proven formula for weight loss (45–30–25) and what you've already consumed that day and that week. You will be given freebies in the following macronutrient groups.

Carbohydrates

This group includes grains and starches (G&S), fruits, non-starchy vegetables (NSV), and milk and milk substitutes. Carbohydrates are the macronutrients our bodies need in the largest quantity. They are the body's main food source and regulate proper functioning of the central nervous system, kidneys, brain, red blood cells, and muscles. They control energy storage in the liver and muscles as well as intestinal health and elimination.

Grains and Starches

Grains and starches are carbohydrates, which include pastas, breads, rice, cereals, and beans. This group also includes starchy vegetables, like potatoes, peas, corn, sweet potatoes, and yams. When it comes to grains, variation is the key. Mix it up and try less-common options like farro and quinoa. Quinoa is relatively new to the United States, but it's been a staple of the Peruvian diet for more than five thousand years. Because of its energy-boosting, high-protein quotient, it was treated like gold by the Incas, who traded it as one of their most precious commodities. Some of the best grains and starches include:

- Brown rice
- Farro
- Quinoa
- Steel cut oats
- Sweet potatoes

As a general rule, the serving size for one G&S portion is one-half cup of cooked pasta, rice, starchy vegetable, or any other grain. A single serving for cold cereals is three-quarters of a cup, and for breads it is about one ounce or usually one slice.

Eating Free highly encourages carbohydrate intake, especially whole grains. You may have heard that whole grains are good for our health and can reduce the risk of many diseases, such as coronary heart disease, obesity, and diabetes. But what are whole grains and how are they beneficial? Whole grains are grains that contain the entire grain seed or kernel, which is made up of three components: bran, germ, and endosperm. If grain has been cracked, crushed, or flaked, the proportions of the original grain must stay about the same. Bran is the outer layer of the grain. It is the tough skin that protects the kernel from the elements. The bran contains B vitamins, fiber, and many important antioxidants. Germ is the part of the grain that is considered to be the embryo. The germ can sprout into a new plant. The germ portion of the grain contains many B vitamins, some proteins, minerals, and healthy fats. Endosperm is the food supply of the grain. It is the largest portion of the kernel and provides the nutrients needed for the plant's survival. The endosperm contains starchy carbohydrates, proteins, and small amounts of vitamins and minerals.

The difference between whole grains and refined grains is that whole grains include all three parts of the grain, while refined grains do not include the bran or germ (these are removed during processing, leaving only the endosperm). With the removal of the bran and germ, 25 percent of the grain's protein and about seventeen key nutrients are lost. I recommend that you consume a variety of G&S throughout the week to optimize your nutritional intake, so mix up your diet with wheat, quinoa, brown rice, and more. For example, if you have cereal for breakfast, maybe add quinoa or beans at lunch and sweet potatoes at dinner.

Grains and Starches	Serving Size	Freebies
Barley, grits, oatmeal, pasta (whole grain, rice, quinoa), rice (brown, white)	½ cup cooked	1 G&S (grains)
Quinoa, farro	½ cup cooked	1.5 G&S + 0.5 meat (grains)
Cold cereal	¾ cup	1 G&S (grains)
Couscous, millet	⅓ cup cooked	1 G&S (grains)
Corn, peas, potato (white, yam, sweet, plain)	½ cup cooked	1 G&S (starchy vegetables)
Squash (winter, butternut, pumpkin)	1 cup cooked	1 G&S (starchy vegetables)
Beans (black, cannellini, garbanzo, kidney, lima), lentils	½ cup cooked	1 G&S + 0.5 meat (legumes)
English muffin, hamburger bun, hot dog bun, 6-inch diameter pita (whole grain, white)	½ piece (1 oz.)	1 G&S (breads)
Bread (corn, whole grain, white, rice, rye)	1 slice (1 oz.)	1 G&S (breads)
Tortilla (whole grain, corn, flour)	5-inch diameter	1 G&S (breads)
Crackers (whole grain, rice), pretzels	0.75 to 1 oz.	1 G&S
Popcorn, air-popped	3 cups	1 G&S

Fruits

Fruits are a good source of carbohydrates and also contain many vitamins, minerals, phytochemicals, and antioxidants. As a general rule, the serving size of fruit is:

½ cup cut fruit

¾ to 1 cup of berries

1 medium-size piece of fruit

2 tablespoons of dried fruit

When it comes to choosing fruits and veggies, I like to tell people to "Eat the rainbow," which means mixing it up with as many colors as you can: red, green, yellow, purple, and orange. Different colors of fruit provide a wide range of vitamins, minerals, fiber, phytochemicals, and antioxidants that your body uses to help maintain a healthy weight, protect against the effects of aging, and reduce the risk of heart disease, type 2 diabetes, high blood pressure, and certain types of cancer. The ideal goal is to eat one of each color in the space of a week, mixing between fruits and vegetables. Think blueberries, bananas, red peppers, squash, and so on. This is important because each color packs different phytonutrients that bring specific benefits. When people tell me all they eat is turkey and broccoli, it makes me nuts. Not only will they get bored and end up bingeing, they're also denying themselves the health perks and satisfaction that come from eating a wide variety of foods prepared in a variety of ways.

Remember to buy your produce in season and, if possible, from a local farmer's market. I suggest this because you'll get the freshest, best-tasting, affordable options available to you. However, I'm not a produce snob, so if you need to eat frozen fruits and veggies to get your quota, then do it. The point is, be sure you're eating nature's bounty one way or another.

Tips on how to increase your fruit intake:

- Add fruit to yogurt.
- Eat a snack.
- Add fruit to cereals.
- Add frozen or fresh fruit to waffles or pancakes.
- Make fruit smoothies.

Non-starchy Vegetables

Non-starchy vegetables (NSV) are a good source of fiber and they contain many vitamins, minerals, phytochemicals, and antioxidants, plus they are very low in calories.

As a general rule, the serving size of one serving of NSV is:

½ cup of raw, cooked, or frozen vegetables
3 cups of raw, leafy vegetables

As with fruits, getting a colorful variety of NSV is important for getting beneficial vitamins, minerals, fiber, phytochemicals, and antioxidants. Some ways to include vegetables in your diet:

- Keep cleaned/prepped veggies in your fridge.
- Double up on veggies in sandwiches/wraps.
- Eat a salad with lunch and dinner, or even as a snack.
- Make stir-fries (add a sauce to diced meat and frozen cut veggies).
- Add extra veggies to sauces and casseroles (like adding carrots to spaghetti sauce).
- Make vegetable soup or get a can of low-sodium soup and add veggies.

- Dip veggies in low-fat salad dressing.
- Add vegetables to side dishes like rice or beans.
- Add vegetables to egg white scrambles.
- Grill or roast zucchini, portabellas, onions, green onions, eggplant, broccoli, cauliflower, brussels sprouts, peppers, or asparagus with a teaspoon of olive oil.

Milk and Milk Substitutes

Milk, soy milk, and yogurt are great sources of protein and calcium. The milk and soy milk group is divided according to fat content. There are four categories of milk: nonfat, 1% milk, 2% milk, and whole milk. Cheese does not contain carbohydrates, so it is listed under the meat food group. Creams and other fatty dairy products are listed as fats. For those with lactose intolerance, look for lactose-free products in all the above categories.

The milk group also includes yogurt. The category is nutritionally important for both protein and calcium, but that doesn't mean you have to have dairy. If you are lactose intolerant, feel free to substitute lactose-free milk, soy milk, almond milk, or rice milk. Just be aware that those milks have only one gram of protein, while a serving of milk has eight grams of protein, so you may need to add protein. Learn your foods and make the decision about whether you want to get your fats from your milk option or if you'd rather save them for a sweet something. If you're like me, you'll opt for low-fat or nonfat milk so you can enjoy your allotted freebie fats in something more exciting than milk.

Food Item	Serving Size	Freebies
Low-fat 1% or nonfat milk, Low-fat 1% or nonfat soy milk, Low-fat 1% or nonfat evaporated milk	1 cup, 8 fluid oz.	1 Milk
Low-fat or nonfat plain yogurt	6 oz.	1 Milk
Low-fat or nonfat plain Greek yogurt	6 oz.	0.5 Milk + 2 Meat
2% milk, 2% soy milk	1 cup, 8 fluid oz.	1 Milk + 1 Fat
Whole milk, goat's milk, kefir	1 cup, 8 fluid oz.	1 Milk + 1.5 Fat
Whole plain yogurt	6 oz.	1 Milk + 1.5 Fat

When it comes to yogurts, types come in plain and natural, sugared, light varieties with artificial sweeteners, and Greek yogurt, which I personally recommend for its probiotics, high protein, and low sugar content. It's a great snack for breakfast or anytime. Just add some fruit and you're good to go.

Proteins

Most Americans get plenty of protein, which is essential for growth, tissue repair, and immune function. Protein also preserves lean muscle mass and helps make essential hormones and enzymes, as well as energy, when carbs aren't available. Proteins are found in meats and vegetarian meats.

Meats and Vegetarian Proteins

Meats and vegetarian meats contain protein and fat. Some meats are fattier than others, and varieties break down into very lean meats, lean meats, medium-fat meats, and high-fat meats.

❑ 1 oz. of meat, poultry, fish, or cheese provide one meat freebie

❑ ½ cup of tofu provides one meat freebie

❏ ½ cup of beans, lentils, quinoa, and farro provide one-half serving of meat (some proteins for the day come from milk or G&S)

As a general rule, I suggest choosing very lean meats most of the time and choosing lean meat some of the time. When consuming lean meat, make heart-healthy choices like salmon, tuna, and tofu. Limit your intake of medium- and high-fat meats as much as you can.

Meats and Vegetarian Meats	Serving Size	Freebies
Beef (ground 4% or 5% fat, extra lean steak, top round), extra lean pork	1 oz.	1 Meat
Chicken or turkey (white meat w/no skin, bacon 95% fat free, ground 4% or 5% fat), Cornish hen (no skin); deli meats, hot dogs, and sausages (with 1 gram of fat or less per ounce)	1 oz.	1 Meat
Fresh or frozen cod, flounder, haddock, halibut, trout, lox (smoked salmon), tuna (fresh or canned in water), clams, crab, lobster, scallops, shrimp, imitation shellfish	1 oz.	1 Meat
Cheese (low-fat or nonfat cottage cheese or ricotta cheese)	¼ cup	1 Meat
Cheese with 1 gram of fat or less per ounce (shredded cheddar, Swiss, American)	1 oz.	1 Meat
Egg (whites, substitute), tofu (lite; less than 2g fat)	¼ cup (egg), 2.8 oz. (tofu)	1 Meat
Beef (trimmed of fat: round, sirloin, flank steak, tenderloin, ground, 7% fat), roast (rib, chuck, rump), steak (T-bone, porterhouse, cubed), veal (lean chop, roast), lamb (roast, chop, or leg), pork (ham, Canadian bacon, tenderloin, center loin chop)	1 oz.	1 Meat + 0.5 Fat
Cheese, 75% reduced fat, 3g fat or less per ounce (grated parmesan, light string cheese, lite creamy cheese)	1 oz.	1 Meat + 0.5 Fat
Chicken (white meat with skin, dark meat without fat and skin, ground 7% fat), salmon, turkey (dark meat without skin, ground 7% fat), deli meat (3g fat or less per ounce)	1 oz.	1 Meat + 0.5 Fat

Meats and Vegetarian Meats *(con't)*	Serving Size	Freebies
Beef (corned, ground beef, 15% fat, prime rib, rib eye, short ribs), veal cutlet, lamb (roast, ground 15% fat), pork (chop, cutlet, top loin chop)	1 oz.	1 Meat + 1 Fat
Cheese, 50% reduced fat (feta, mozzarella, Jarlsberg, string cheese)	1 oz.	1 Meat + 1 Fat
Chicken or turkey (dark meat w/skin, ground 15% fat), Fried chicken or fish	1 oz.	1 Meat + 1 Fat
Edamame (soy beans), tofu (regular 5g fat per 4 ounces), whole egg (hard-boiled, scrambled, poached, fried), tempeh	½ cup (edamame & tofu), 1 egg, ¼ cup (tempeh)	1 Meat + 1 Fat
Beef (brisket, spareribs), pork (ground, spareribs, bacon), sausage, hot dogs, and deli meat (8g fat per ounce)	1 oz.	1 Meat + 2 Fat
Cheese, regular, 8g fat per ounce (Monterey Jack, cheddar, brie)	1 oz.	1 Meat + 2 Fat
Peanut butter (smooth, crunchy)	2 tablespoons	1 Meat + 2 Fat

My biggest rule for meats, which allows people to eat what they enjoy most, is to stay with lean meats whenever possible. They have fewer saturated fats, which cause inflammation that leads to a host of diseases. The trick is to check the meats you buy for fat content. Many dieters only eat chicken and turkey, which can get boring fast. But guess what: if you buy lean red meat, you can enjoy that too. I always look for a label that says "less than 4% fat" or "96% lean" on my beef. Then I feel free to make burgers, spaghetti sauce, whatever I'm craving. As I mentioned, you're going to be given some freebie fats for each week, divided into daily amounts, but if you're eating full-fat meats and dairy, you'll use those credits up instead of adding a heart-healthy fat like avocado onto your burger.

Learn the Fat Contents of Various Kinds of Meat

Very Lean (0–4% fat). This isn't a category comprised solely of bland chicken. Within this group, you'll also find pork loin chops, pork tenderloin, beef, turkey breast, and even some low-fat chicken or turkey sausages. If you don't see any cuts with this low percentage in the meat case, have your butcher grind sirloin steak—a naturally lean cut—and you're good to go.

Lean (7–10% fat). This group includes dark chicken, steaks, and salmon, which we love because it's rich in omega-3s. It's a great idea to have 6–8 ounces of wild salmon per week. If it's not in season, try using canned salmon instead of tuna. I make a great canned salmon salad, and you can find the recipe in Chapter 12, "Freecipes."

Medium fat (up to 15%). This is the highest fat-content beef, and what we typically purchase just because we may not read the label. I often hear that my clients believe grass-fed beef is leaner, but they are sadly mistaken.

High fat. This group includes decadent foods like cheeses, bacon, sausage, and more. While you can enjoy them without fear, you should allow them in moderation.

Fats

Although fats have a bad reputation for causing weight gain, some fats are essential for survival. We need fats for normal growth and development, energy, absorption of vitamins A, D, E, K, and carotenoids, as well as for the cushioning of organs. Fats are found in:

- Butter
- Fish
- Grain products

- Lard
- Margarines
- Meat
- Milk
- Nuts
- Oils
- Poultry

Please note that there are three kinds of fats: saturated fats (found in meat, butter, lard, tropical oils, and cream), unsaturated fats (found in olive oil, avocados, nuts, salmon, and canola oil), and trans fats (found in baked goods, snack foods, fried foods, and margarines). While it's important to know that replacing saturated and trans fats with "good fats" has been shown to decrease your risk of developing heart disease and inflammation, eating "good fats" does not necessarily lend itself to weight loss. You are required to eat fats while Eating Free, and I always recommend the "good" ones for health reasons. However, fats are fats and they need to be consumed within the 45–30–25 formula to help you achieve and maintain weight loss. Just because they are "good" fats doesn't mean they can be consumed freely while trying to lose weight.

This group includes foods that contain a significant amount of healthy fats, including oils such as olive and coconut oil, nuts, flaxseeds, and avocados. The way many of us eat, we make burgers with full-fat beef, add cheese, and then avocado as well. On the Eating Free plan, I'll teach you to enjoy that same burger, made with lean beef, topped with the proper serving of avocado, and a low-fat cheese.

You see, most people are eating their heart-healthy, "good for you" fats but *also* eating full-fat beef burgers without even thinking about it. Still other people eat their burgers without a bun because they've sworn off carbs. But your freebies give you a grain allotment. So eat a lean beef burger on a whole grain bun with avocado on top and you've got nothing to worry about. You've created the taste you crave while eating things you can feel great about—and you will still lose weight!

Fat is an important and necessary part of our diets; we cannot survive without it. Some of the health benefits of fat include: energy storage, breakdown of fat-soluble vitamins and phytonutrients, and hormone synthesis. However, certain fats are more beneficial than others; not all fats were created equal. "Bad" fats include trans fat (which comes from partially hydrogenated oils). They are dubbed bad fats because they are known to contribute to cardiovascular disease. This is why it is very important to reduce your consumption of these fats and instead focus on monounsaturated and polyunsaturated fats, including omega-3s and omega-6s. These fats are anti-inflammatory and prevent chronic diseases, and they have been proven to be beneficial for your body. If there is one fat I recommend avoiding as much as possible, it's hydrogenated fats. They have no value and do demonstrable harm.

Saturated Fats	Monounsat. Fats	Omega-6	Omega-3	Trans Fat
Butter	Canola oil	Safflower oil	Walnuts	Margarines
Cream	Olive oil	Sunflower oil	Flaxseeds	Packaged foods prepared with hydrogenated oils
Whole-fat cheeses	Almonds	Corn oil	Soybeans	Fast foods
Sausages	Avocado	Sesame oil	Salmon	
Bacon	Olives	Pumpkin oil	Sardines	
Fatty red meat	Cashews	Soybean oil	Mackerel	
Whole milk	Pistachios		Hemp seeds	
Palm, coconut oil			Walnut oil	

Fats	Serving Size	Freebies
Avocado	2 tablespoons	1 Fat
Butter, margarine (stick, tub, squeeze), mayonnaise (regular)	1 teaspoon	1 Fat
Flaxseed (ground), salad dressing (reduced fat)	2 tablespoons	1 Fat
Mayonnaise (reduced fat), Miracle Whip salad dressing (reduced fat), salad dressing (regular)	1 teaspoon	1 Fat
Nuts (almonds, cashews, pecans, walnuts)	4–6 nuts	1 Fat
Nuts (peanuts, pistachios)	10–15 nuts	1 Fat
Oils (canola, olive, peanut, hazelnut, corn, safflower, soybean, grapeseed, walnut)	1 teaspoon	1 Fat
Olives (black, green stuffed)	8–10 large	1 Fat
Whole seeds (pumpkin, sunflower, sesame, flaxseed)	1 tablespoon	1 Fat

In addition to the three main macronutrient groups, there are other groups that will be part of your program. They are not required foods, but they are allowed, and you will learn how to plug them into your food program and monitor their consumption.

Combination Foods

There are also combination groups for foods like pizza and sushi. These are foods that effectively combine more than one freebie into their mix. Certain meats are combinations, like bacon, for example, which contains meat and fat.

Combination foods are foods that do not fit exactly into one food group. As the name implies, they are combinations of different food groups, as well as food group allowances. The following table has some examples of combination foods. Your online food record will have a more complete list.

Food Item	Serving Size	Freebies
Beef stew	1 cup (8 fl. oz.)	1.5 G&S + 2 Meat + 1 NSV + 2 Fat
Burrito (w/chicken, beans, cheese, guacamole, sour cream)	13-inch (9 oz.)	3.5 G&S + 4 Meat + 5 Fat
Chef salad	1 cup	3 Meat + 0.5 NSV + 2.5 Fat
Chicken teriyaki w/rice	1 meal	2.5 G&S + 4 Meat + 2 Fat + 2 Sugar
Chili	1 cup (8 oz.)	2 G&S + 2 Meat + 2 Fat
Chips, tortilla or potato	9-13 pieces	1 G&S + 1 Fat
French fries	1 medium (5 oz.)	4 G&S + 4 Fat
Fried chicken	3 pieces (4.6 oz.)	2 G&S + 3 Meat + 3.5 Fat
Fried rice	1 cup (5 oz.)	2 G&S + 2 Fat
Grilled cheese sandwich	1 sandwich	2 G&S + 1 Meat + 4 Fat
Hamburger, Quarter Pounder, no cheese	1 quarter pounder (6 oz.)	2.3 G&S + 5 Meat + 5 Fat
Meat lasagna	1 cup (8 oz.)	2 G&S + 2 Meat + 2 Fat
Pizza, cheese, thin crust	¼ of 12-inch (5 oz.)	2 G&S + 2 Meat + 2 Fat
Pizza, meat topping, thin crust	¼ of 12-inch (5 oz.)	2 G&S + 2 Meat + 3.5 Fat
Soft chicken taco	1 taco	2 G&S + 2 Meat + 3 Fat
Spaghetti w/meatballs	1 cup	2 G&S + 2 Meat + 2 Fat
Stir-fry w/meat & vegetables	1 cup	4 Meat + 2 NSV + 3 Fat + 3 Sugar
Sushi, California roll	6 pieces	2 G&S + 1 Meat + 1 Fat
Tempura, vegetable	5 pieces, variety	1 G&S + 2 NSV + 3 Fat
Veggie sandwich, no cheese, no mayo	1 sandwich (6-inch)	2 G&S + 1 Meat + 1 NSV + 1 Fat

Sugars

My plan always encourages moderation. However, as a general rule, the Eating Free program doesn't always allocate sugar freebies. You will decide how to proceed with sugar based on your calorie level, exercise level, and preferences. You could meet your caloric levels by eating sugars, but you may not have yet eaten the whole foods—like grains and fruits—that your body needs to lose weight. You need to stick to your optimal deficit, but if you meet your goal by just eating sugars, you'll get hungry and frustrated, which can lead to a binge. (The online tracking will teach you what whole foods you need, and in what amounts, so you can be successful.) I'm not saying to skip sugars entirely, just to learn how to add them to your plan without derailing your progress.

Added sugars that supply extra calories to your diet need to be monitored. They can come from packaged foods and sweeteners, like syrups, honey, agave, molasses, high fructose corn syrup, corn syrup, cane juice, and table sugar. You can find the type of added sugar in packaged foods listed in the ingredients, which are posted in descending order from most to least. If the first ingredient is a sugar, then the main type of carbohydrate is from sugar. Sugars don't provide many vitamins, minerals, phytochemicals, or antioxidants. They are considered "empty calories," void of nutritional value. I recommend that no more than 10 percent of your total calories come from added sugars.

Naturally occurring sugars like fructose in fruits and lactose in milk are not counted as "sugar" in your plan because they are associated with foods that are nutrient-dense. Plus, the benefits of eating fruit and milk products outweigh the negative effects of the sugar they contain.

An example of the difference between naturally occurring sugar and added sugar is plain yogurt versus flavored yogurt. Plain yogurt contains lactose-based sugars, which equal about 12 grams of carbohydrates. But if you add fruit flavor to the yogurt, the amount of carbohydrates per serving can almost triple to 30 grams. These extra amounts of carbohydrates come from added sugars and add extra calories to your daily intake.

So let's talk about how to incorporate sugars responsibly. Is having a sweet tooth okay, or should you fight it at all costs? The truth is that a sweet tooth is tough to fight! Think about it. Our first craving from birth is sugar, delivered to us as infants via our mother's milk. Our first meal is a sweet meal! So why wouldn't we crave sugar for life?

A sweet tooth, for the purpose of this topic, is defined as wanting something sweet after your meal. That's why it's important to make sure that you eat all of your meals so that you don't confuse a sweet tooth with real hunger, which can make you crave sugars. I firmly believe there's nothing wrong with having a sweet tooth. I grew up having a nice home-made dessert as part of a healthy, balanced meal, and I have developed a good relationship with my sweet tooth. You may feel guilty about sugar cravings and feel pressured to fight temptation to indulge, but this only sets you up to binge later on. You really should just allow yourself to have a reasonable amount of a sensible, sweet snack. Celebrate your sweet tooth. Just don't forget to practice portion control!

Here are some ideas that will satisfy your sweet tooth and your diet:

- ❏ Two to three pieces of dark chocolate (at least 70 percent cocoa)
- ❏ Three dried figs plus one piece of dark chocolate (my personal favorite)
- ❏ Strawberries with light whipped cream
- ❏ Greek yogurt (nonfat, plain) with one tablespoon of fruit preserves (no sugar added) or one tablespoon honey

Dessert Food Item	Serving Size	Freebies
Bread pudding w/caramel sauce	1 (5.7 oz.)	1.3 G&S, 0.5 Meat , 5 Fat, 1.7 Sugar
Cake (frosted), cupcake	2 oz.	1 G&S + 1 Fat + 1 Sugar
Cake, unfrosted	1 oz.	1 G&S + 1 Fat
Cake, cheese	1 slice (6.7 oz.)	1 G&S + 1.5 Meat + 9 Fat + 3 Sugar
Cake, carrot	1 slice (4.5 oz.)	2 G&S + 5.5 Fat + 2.5 Sugar
Cake, chocolate	1 slice (2.3 oz.)	1 G&S + 2 Fat + 1.5 Sugar
Chocolate bar, milk	1 oz. (28g)	2.5 Fat + 1.5 Sugar
Chocolate bar, 73% dark	1 oz. (28g)	2 Fat + 0.5 Sugar
Cookie (chocolate chip, oatmeal, peanut butter, sugar)	1 cookie (3 oz.)	2 G&S + 4 Fat + 2 Sugar
Doughnut, glazed	1 medium (1.5-2 oz.)	1 G&S + 1 Fat + 1 Sugar
Fruit crisp or cobbler	½ cup	1 G&S + 1 Fruit + 1 Fat
Ice cream	½ cup	1 Milk + 3.5 Fat
Ice cream, low-fat	½ cup	1 Milk + 1 Fat + 1 Sugar
Pie (apple, sweet potato)	⅛ of 9-inch pie	1.5 G&S + 2.5 Fat + 1.5 Sugar
Pie (lemon meringue, pecan)	1/6 of 8-inch pie	1.5 G&S + 3 Fat + 1.5 Sugar
Pudding, rice	½ cup	0.5 G&S + 0.5 Milk + 0.5 Fat + 0.5 Sugar
Pudding, regular (chocolate, vanilla, banana)	½ cup	0.5 Milk + 0.5 Fat + 1 Sugar
Rice Krispies treat	1 bar	0.5 G&S, 0.5 Fat, 0.5 Sugar
Sherbet, sorbet	½ cup	2 Sugars
Yogurt, frozen, regular	⅓ cup	1 Fat + 1 Sugar
Yogurt, frozen, nonfat	⅓ cup	1 Sugar
Agave nectar, honey, syrup	1 tablespoon	1 Sugar

Dessert Food Item	Serving Size	Freebies
Barbeque sauce	1 tablespoon	1 Sugar
Jam, jelly, regular	1 tablespoon	1 Sugar
Ketchup	3 tablespoons	1 Sugar

Alcohol

Drinking alcohol is definitely a choice that only you alone can make. As stated before, I believe that moderation is key, so if you do drink alcohol, it can be worked into your plan. However, I recommend consuming no more than four servings of alcohol per week for weight loss.

You may be surprised to learn that, from a nutritional standpoint, alcohol will count as a fat. This is not because alcohol itself has a fat content. It's because when your liver is processing alcohol, it cannot process fat—it only does one function at a time. So the fact that you're not metabolizing fat when you're drinking means you're holding on to fats that would otherwise be processed. For that reason, when you choose to drink alcohol, it counts as if you ate a fat. This simple piece of knowledge has helped a number of my clients decide how to wisely integrate alcohol while trying to lose weight.

Many people enjoy a glass of wine with dinner as a matter of course, or because they are foodies. But once they learn that the glass of wine counts as extra fat every dinnertime, they don't hesitate to drop that habit. They choose, instead, to enjoy wine when at restaurants or on weekends or once a week. This is the kind of decision I refer to as making policies about food. I don't say, "Quit drinking wine." I arm you with the knowledge that when your body is processing it, you may as well be eating fats. Once you know that, you are empowered to decide what's more important: shedding the weight or enjoying the wine. The great thing is, once you achieve your goal weight, you'll be able to reintroduce things like wine with more regularity because you'll be on a maintenance plan rather than a weight-loss program.

For weight loss, there's no specific research, but what I've observed is that men may have six to seven servings per week, while women may have four to five servings per week. Now mind you, a serving is four ounces of wine, a shot of booze, or twelve ounces of beer. And remember, the oversized globe wineglasses in restaurants contain six ounces a pour (one and a half servings). A glass of wine in your house usually equals eight ounces (two servings). Cocktails in restaurants may include two shots and equal two servings. Some information to consider about alcohol is listed below.

Serving Sizes

The amount of alcohol a person can drink safely depends on the type of alcohol they consume. Generally, a serving size is considered to be: four ounces of wine, ten ounces of a wine cooler, twelve ounces of beer, or one and a half ounces of distilled liquor. If you are not trying to lose weight, the National Institute of Health recommends that women drink no more than one serving size per day and men no more than two (this is recommended only if you are not pregnant, lactating, have alcohol dependencies, diseases, or are taking medications that interact negatively with alcohol).

Cons of Alcohol for Weight Regulation and Other Health Risks

Alcohol is a toxin (poison), and because of this the body absorbs and metabolizes it as quickly as possible to ensure a fast exit. The effects of alcohol can be felt almost instantaneously: it takes as little as one minute to reach the brain.

- Alcohol stimulates appetite, which puts you at risk for higher calorie intake. Alcohol also lowers your inhibitions, making it easier to choose unhealthy foods.

- Numerous studies have concluded that alcohol can also increase your risk of numerous types of cancer, accidental death due to judgment impairment (the number one cause of death in the United States), miscarriage, having a child with fetal alcohol syndrome, and heart muscle damage.

- Alcohol can also have seriously negative effects on your body if you are taking antibiotics, anticoagulants, antidepressants, diabetes medications, beta blockers, pain relievers, or sleeping pills.

Drink Item	Serving Size	Freebies
Beer	12 oz.	1 G&S + 2 Fat
Light beer	12 oz.	2 Fat
Champagne	4 oz.	2 Fat
Cocktail (cosmopolitan, mojito)	4 oz.	2 Fat + 1 Sugar
Hard liquor (whiskey, vodka, tequila, rum)	1.5 oz.	2 Fat
Margarita	5 oz.	2 Fat + 3 Sugar
Sangria	4 oz.	2 Fat + 1 Sugar
Wine (red, white)	4 oz.	2 Fat
Wine, dessert	4 oz.	2 Fat + 2 Sugar

Healthy Eating Does Not Equal Weight Loss

Many clients arrive at my office and tell me, "I have cut out all processed food. I eat all organically and I mainly eat salmon and olive oil, but I'm not losing weight." I tell them they may be organically growing their waistline.

It's important to note that, within any category, a serving is a serving. So many of my clients confuse heart-healthy foods with foods for weight loss. That is to say, a half cup of brown rice is the same as a half cup of white rice when it comes to measuring portions for weight loss. Will the brown rice pack more power in terms of fiber and other benefits? Absolutely! But will it make you lose weight faster? No. And can you eat more of it because it's healthier? No. This is an essential concept to grasp, because so many people assume that eating heart-healthy foods like salmon, olive oil, avocado, brown rice, and sweet potatoes means free rein to eat unlimited portions. I can't tell you how many times I hear clients say, "I ate a whole avocado, but it's okay because it's a good fat." *Listen up:* A fat is a fat is a fat. It's all about portions, no matter how heart-healthy, low-fat, organic, gluten-free, or low-carb that food may be.

> It's all about portions, no matter how heart-healthy, low-fat, organic, gluten-free, or low-carb that food may be.

With your freebies, you will be allotted a certain number of fats per week—and you can eat them from whatever whole, real foods you like. Of course, I would prefer you get your fats from an avocado rather than from mayonnaise, but the fat measurement is the same. Just think how many times you've allowed yourself more brown rice or more salmon because it's so healthy. It is indeed healthy, but it still counts in the equation when you're eating to lose weight. This is why understanding portion sizes is so critical.

Below are some of the top foods that are healthy, but still can't be eaten in unlimited quantities while trying to lose weight:

Brown Rice: Nutritionally speaking, brown rice is better than white— it has more fiber and it's a whole grain, but that doesn't mean you get to eat more of it. Once you learn that the proper serving size is a half cup, you must recognize that the measurement applies to all kinds of rice.

Olive Oil: Olive oil is another ingredient people allow themselves in ample quantities because they know it is a healthy fat. However, one teaspoon is the proper serving size, not liberal pours from the bottle.

Avocado: Here again, people understand that this is a healthy food choice, but it is still a fat. The proper serving size for an avocado is about one-eighth of the fruit.

Almonds: Nuts make a great snack, but you can't just eat them by the handful. The proper serving size is approximately six nuts.

Salmon: I am a big advocate of salmon, and I recommend all of my clients eat it at least once a week for the omega-3s. However, salmon is not as lean as other types of proteins, so it's something you should learn to eat in the proper portion sizes.

100% Fruit Juices: Juices are packed with antioxidants, but a serving size is only a mere four fluid ounces not twenty-four ounces.

Your Seven-Day Sample Meal Plans and Recipes

In order for you to see how freebies work with real foods, I am providing you with four different daily caloric levels: 1,200, 1,400, 1,800, and 2,100—the four most popular levels of calories I see in my practice. Find the one that works for you. Each plan follows proper freebie components in the 45–30–25 formula. And while I have easy online tools to find your custom program, you can also figure out exactly what you need using the tables provided below. *Please note:* These menus don't serve as a diet. These are merely suggested meals that follow the 45–30–25 formula so you can begin to learn how to put together appropriate meals in the optimal Eating Free combinations. There are four typical meal plans in which freebies are broken into nutritional groups and portioned. Because everyone's weight-loss prescription is so customized, I recommend using my free online tool (at www.eatingfree.com) to calculate your optimal deficit and then find the nearest caloric menu here. So, for example, if your optimal deficit comes to 1,700 calories a day, follow the 1,800-calories-a-day recommendation. However, if you're not able to access the online tool, I've included a paper format as well, so you'll be able to begin Eating Free solely using this book. Some of the recipes are used in my sample menus, but I've also provided other examples in the meal plans so you can understand how to use real foods to achieve your goals.

Here are some tips to help you decide which caloric meal plan you may want to follow if you don't go online:

- **1,200-Calorie Meal Plan:** Developed for the average female age fifty to sixty-five years old with a sedentary or light activity desk job, this plan assumes the reader dose not exercise or exercises one to two days per week. If you exercise vigorously (running, circuit training, spinning) more than three days per week, then follow the 1,400-calorie plan.

- **1,400-Calorie Meal Plan:** Developed for the average female age twenty to forty-nine years old with a sedentary or light activity desk job, this plan assumes you exercise two to three days per week. If you exercise vigorously (running, circuit training, spinning) more than three days per week, please calculate your prescription by visiting www.eatingfree.com. If you begin with the 1,400-calorie meal plan and aren't losing weight, then follow the 1,200-calorie plan.

- **1,800-Calorie Meal Plan:** Developed for the average male age fifty to sixty-five years old with a sedentary or light activity desk job, this plan assumes that you do not exercise or exercise one to two days per week. If you exercise vigorously (running, circuit training, spinning) more than three days per week, then follow the 2,100-calorie plan.

- **2,100-Calorie Meal Plan:** Developed for the average male age twenty to forty-nine years old with a sedentary or light activity desk job, this plan assumes you exercise two to three days per week. If you exercise vigorously (running, circuit training, spinning) more than three days per week, please calculate your prescription by visiting www.eatingfree.com. If you begin with the 2,100-calorie meal plan and don't lose weight, then follow the 1,800-calorie plan.

I have also summarized the freebies for other calorie levels using the 45–30–25 formula in the following table. You can decide on your freebies based on the freebies form in the meal plan provided.

Calories	G&S	Fruit	NSV	Milk	Meat	Fat	Carbohydrate grams	Protein grams	Fat grams
1200	4	3	4	1	9	4	137	91	32
1300	4	3	4	2	9	5	149	99	39
1400	5	3	5	2	9	5	168	104	40
1500	5	3	5	2	10	6	168	111	44
1600	5	4	5	2	11	6	184	118	46
1700	5	4	5	2	13	6	184	132	48
1800	6	4	5	2	14	6	199	142	50
1900	7	4	5	2	14	7	214	145	56
2000	7	4	6	2	15	7	219	154	56
2100	7	4	6	3	15	7	231	162	58
2200	8	5	6	3	15	7	261	165	58

1,200 Calorie Food Plan: *Day 1*

AMOUNT		FREEBIES	INSTRUCTIONS
BREAKFAST	**Banana Walnut Steel Cut Oatmeal**		
1 serving	*Banana Walnut Steel Cut Oatmeal*	1 G&S, 1 Meat, 1 Fat	*See recipe list.*
2 Tbsp.	Flaxseed meal	1 Fat	Add flaxseed
¾ cup	Blueberries	1 Fruit	meal and blue-
1 cup	Low-fat 1% or nonfat milk	1 Milk	berries to oatmeal
		355 calories	after warming up. Serve milk on the side.
SNACK	**Cheese & Crackers**		
1½ oz.	Lite creamy cheese	1 Meat, 0.5 Fat	
1 oz.	Whole grain or rice crackers	1 G&S	
		135 calories	
LUNCH	**Turkey Pita Pocket**		
½	Whole grain pita pocket	1 G&S	Stuff pita with
½ cup	Non-starchy mixed vegetables such as lettuce, tomato, sprouts, pepperoncini	1 NSV	mixed vegetables, turkey, and avocado. Enjoy
1 oz.	Turkey deli slice	1 Meat	baby carrots on
2 Tbsp.	Avocado	1 Fat	the side.
15	Baby carrots	1 NSV	
		210 calories	
SNACK	**Veggie & Hummus Platter**		
1 cup	Celery sticks, baby carrots, bell peppers (sliced)	1 NSV	*See recipe list.*
¼ cup	*Zesty Hummus*	1 G&S, 0.5 Meat, 0.5 Fat	
		145 calories	
DINNER	**Fish and Rice**		
1 serving	*Thai Soy Cilantro Fish*	4 Meat, 0.5 Fat	*See recipe list.*
½ cup	Steamed jasmine rice	1 G&S	Spray asparagus
8	Asparagus spears	1 NSV	lightly with olive
1 spray	Oil	Free	oil and roast
		268 calories	alongside fish for 10 minutes.
DESSERT	**Dark Chocolate & Dried Figs**		
15 grams	Dark chocolate, 70% or more dark	1 Fat, 1 Sugar	
3	Dried figs	1 Fruit	
		165 calories	

1,200 CALORIE FOOD PLAN: *Day 2*

AMOUNT		FREEBIES	INSTRUCTIONS
BREAKFAST	**Open Face Breakfast a la Med**		
½ muffin	Whole grain English muffin	1 G&S	Toast English
1 Tbsp.	Fat-free cream cheese	Free	muffin, spread
1 oz.	Smoked salmon	1 Meat, 0.5 Fat	cream cheese and
1	Tomato slices	NSV	layer with salmon,
¼ cup	Raw spinach	NSV	tomato and spin-
1 cup	Low-fat 1% or nonfat milk	1 Milk	ach. Serve milk
¾ cup	Pineapple chunks	1 Fruit	and pineapple on
		285 calories	the side.
SNACK	**Cheese & Crackers**		
1 oz.	Low-fat cheese	1 Meat, 0.5 Fat	
1 oz.	Whole grain or rice crackers	1 G&S	
		135 calories	
LUNCH	**Egg Salad Tacos**		
2	Eggs, hard boiled and chopped	2 Meat, 2 Fat	Mix eggs, mus-
1 Tbsp.	Dijon mustard	Free	tard, and shallots
1 small	Shallot, finely diced	1 NSV	together, then
	(alternative: 2 Tbsp. celery)		spread evenly
2 leaves	Romaine lettuce, chopped	NSV	on each tortilla.
2	Corn tortilla 5-inch diameter	2 G&S	Sprinkle lettuce
1 medium	Apple	1 Fruit	evenly on top of
		395 calories	the egg mixture
			and fold. Enjoy
			apple on the side.
SNACK	**Yogurt & Berries**		
6 oz.	Nonfat plain Greek yogurt	2 Meat, 0.5 Milk	
¾ cup	Blueberries	1 Fruit	
		175 calories	
DINNER	**Spaghetti & Meat Sauce**		
½ cup	Whole grain, rice, or quinoa pasta	1 G&S	Cook pasta.
½ cup	Low-fat tomato marinara sauce	2 NSV, 0.5 Fat	Combine browned
2 oz.	Lean ground turkey, browned	2 Meat, 1 Fat	ground turkey
½ cup	Green beans, steamed	1 NSV	with marinara
1 spray	Oil	Free	sauce and heat;
½ Tbsp.	Red wine vinegar	Free	pour over pasta
		293 calories	and top with
			Parmesan. Toss
			green beans in oil
			and vinegar and
			enjoy on the side.

1,200 Calorie Food Plan: *Day 3*

AMOUNT		FREEBIES	INSTRUCTIONS
BREAKFAST	**High Fiber Cereal & Nuts**		
½ cup	High fiber cereal	1 G&S	Mix everything
¾ cup	Blueberries	1 Fruit	in a bowl. It's that
1 cup	Low-fat 1% or nonfat milk	1 Milk	simple.
4	Walnut halves, crushed into small pieces	1 Fat	
		275 calories	
SNACK	**Egg & Apple**		
1	Hard boiled egg	1 Meat, 1 Fat	
1	Small apple, cut into slices	1 Fruit	
		135 calories	
LUNCH	**Smoked Salmon Tea Sandwiches**		
2 slices	Dark rye bread	2 G&S	Layer everything
3 oz.	Smoked salmon	3 Meat	to make a refresh-
2 Tbsp.	Fat-free cream cheese	Free	ing sandwich.
1 Tbsp.	Capers	Free	You can spread
1 slice	Red onion	0.5 NSV	mustard if you
4 thin slices	Tomato	0.5 NSV	want.
4 thin slices	Cucumber	NSV	
		290 calories	
SNACK	**Pineapple Parfait**		
¼ cup	Cottage cheese, nonfat	1 Meat	Mix everything
¾ cup	Pineapple chunks	1 Fruit	together.
		95 calories	
DINNER	**Paprika Chicken & Roasted Vegetables**		
3 oz.	Chicken breast	3 Meat	Sprinkle lemon
1 Tbsp.	Lemon juice	Free	and paprika on
¼ tsp.	Paprika	Free	both sides of
½ cup	Sweet potatoes, baked	1 G&S	chicken. Wrap 1 sweet potato in
1 serving	*Roasted Vegetables*	2 NSV, 0.5 Fat	foil. Bake both
		258 calories	items in oven at 375°F for 20–25 minutes. *See recipe list.*

1,200 CALORIE FOOD PLAN: *Day 4*

AMOUNT		FREEBIES	INSTRUCTIONS
BREAKFAST	Quinoa-Coconut Wake-up Bowl		
½ cup	Quinoa, cooked	1.5 G&S, 0.5 Meat	Mix everything
½ cup	Mango or fruit of choice, cut up	1 Fruit	together. Enjoy
1 Tbsp.	Shredded coconut, sweetened	1 Fat	milk on the side.
1 cup	Low-fat 1% or nonfat milk	1 Milk	
		333 calories	
SNACK	Veggie & Hummus Platter		
1 cup	Celery sticks, baby carrots, bell peppers (sliced)	1 NSV	*See recipe list.*
¼ cup	*Zesty Hummus*	1 G&S, 0.5 Meat, 0.5 Fat	
		145 calories	
LUNCH	No-Mayo Tuna Salad		
3 oz.	Canned tuna in water	3 Meat	Drain the tuna.
1 cup	Cherry tomatoes	1 NSV	Mix tuna and
½ cup	Beans (canned, cooked, or vacuum packed)	1 G&S	everything else together. Serve
3½ cups	Salad mix/baby spinach	1 NSV	pineapple on the
1 Tbsp.	Salad dressing or vinaigrette, light	0.5 Fat	side.
¾ cup	Pineapple chunks	1 Fruit	
		318 calories	
SNACK	Yogurt & Berries		
6 oz.	Nonfat plain Greek yogurt	2 Meat, 0.5 Milk	
¾ cup	Blueberries	1 Fruit	
		175 calories	
DINNER	Meatloaf and Veggies		
1 serving	*Heart Healthy Turkey Meatloaf*	3.5 Meat, 1 NSV, 0.5 Fat	*See recipe list.* Toss broccoli with olive oil and
½ cup	Broccoli, steamed	1 NSV	lemon juice. Serve
1 tsp.	Olive oil	1 Fat	on the side with
1 Tbsp.	Lemon juice	Free	cannellini bean puree.
½ cup	*Tuscan White Bean Puree*	1 G&S, 1 Meat, 0.5 Fat	*See recipe list.*
		378 calories	

1,200 CALORIE FOOD PLAN: *Day 5*

AMOUNT		FREEBIES	INSTRUCTIONS
BREAKFAST	Sausage, Egg, & Tomato Sandwich		
2½ oz.	Chicken sausage link	1.5 Meat, 1 Fat	Assemble every-
1	Egg, whole	1 Meat, 1 Fat	thing together
1 slice	Whole grain, rice, or corn toast	1 G&S	and serve milk on
1 tsp.	Butter (for toast)	1 Fat	the side.
1	Tomato, quartered	1 NSV	
1 cup	Low-fat 1% or nonfat milk	1 Milk	
		413 calories	
SNACK	Sweet Potato & Greek Yogurt		
6 oz.	Nonfat plain Greek yogurt	2 Meat, 0.5 Milk	Use leftover
½ cup	Sweet potato, roasted	1 G&S	sweet potato and
		195 calories	mix with Greek yogurt.
LUNCH	Soup & Ham 'n' Cheese Sandwich		
1 cup	Low-fat tomato soup (made with water)	2 NSV	Heat soup in microwave.
1 slice	Whole grain, rice, or corn toast	1 G&S	Layer ham,
1 oz.	Low-fat cheddar cheese	1 Meat, 0.5 Fat	cheese, and Dijon
1 oz.	Ham, sliced, 99% fat-free	1 Meat	on bread. Enjoy
1 Tbsp.	Dijon mustard	Free	baby carrots and
3	Dried figs	1 Fruit	figs on the side.
15	Baby carrots	1 NSV	
		355 calories	
SNACK	Nuts 'n' Fruit		
4	Walnut halves	1 Fat	
1 medium	Apple	1 Fruit	
		105 calories	
DINNER	Farro and Shrimp		
1 serving	*Farro Roasted Vegetable Salad*	2 G&S, 2 NSV, 1 Meat, 0.5 Fat	*See recipe list.* For shrimp: put
8	Shrimp, medium, to serve on the side	2 Meat	on two skewers, sprinkle with
1 Tbsp.	Lime juice	Free	lime juice and
		338 calories	grill.
DESSERT	Dark Chocolate & Dried Apricots		
15 grams	Dark chocolate, 70% or more dark	1 Fat, 1 Sugar	
5	Dried apricot halves	1 Fruit	
		165 calories	

1,200 CALORIE FOOD PLAN: *Day 6*

AMOUNT		FREEBIES	INSTRUCTIONS
BREAKFAST	**Morning Smoothie**		
4 oz.	Nonfat plain Greek yogurt	1 Meat, 0.3 Milk	Blend everything
½ cup	Low-fat 1% milk or nonfat milk	0.5 Milk	together and
½ cup	Cooked oatmeal	1 G&S	enjoy!
	(or ¼ cup uncooked)		
1¼ cup	Strawberries	1 Fruit	
2 Tbsp.	Flaxseed meal, ground	1 Fat	
		292 calories	
SNACK	**Mango Parfait**		
½ cup	Mango or fruit of choice, cut up	1 Fruit	
¼ cup	Cottage cheese, nonfat	1 Meat	
		95 calories	
LUNCH	**Arugula Salmon Salad**		
½ cup	Whole grain, rice, or quinoa pasta	1 G&S	Mix all ingredients
3 oz.	Canned salmon, water packed,	3 Meat, 1.5 Fat	thoroughly in a
	drained		bowl. Serve pine-
2½ cups	Arugula	1 NSV	apple on the side.
½ lemon	Juice from ½ lemon	Fruit	
1 spray	Oil	Free	
To taste	Dried chili flakes, salt & pepper	Free	
¾ cup	Pineapple	1 Fruit	
		410 calories	
SNACK	**Veggie & Hummus Platter**		
1 cup	Celery sticks, baby carrots,	1 NSV	*See recipe list.*
	bell peppers (sliced)		
¼ cup	*Zesty Hummus*	1 G&S, 0.5 Meat,	
		0.5 Fat	
		145 calories	
DINNER	**Mexican Fiesta Night**		
1 serving	*Spicy Steak Fajitas*	3 Meat, 1.5 Fat, 1 NSV,	*See recipe list.*
		1 G&S	
½ serving	*Roasted Vegetables*	1 NSV, 0.25 Fat	*See recipe list.*
¼ cup	Salsa	0.5 NSV	Top fajita with
		376 calories	salsa.

1,200 Calorie Food Plan: *Day 7*

AMOUNT		FREEBIES	INSTRUCTIONS
BREAKFAST	**French Toast & Strawberries with Sausage**		
1	Egg white, beaten and combined with 1 Tbsp. water	0.5 Meat	Combine egg, water, and vanilla and beat. Dip each slice of bread in the egg mixture and fry in a nonstick pan coated lightly with canola oil (use a sprayer). Top with strawberries and syrup. Serve the chicken sausage link on the side.
1 tsp.	Vanilla extract, added to egg and water		
1 slice	Whole grain, rice, or corn bread	1 G&S	
⅔ cup	Strawberries, sliced	0.5 Fruit	
1 Tbsp.	Maple syrup	1 Sugar	
1 spray	Oil	Free	
2½ oz.	Chicken sausage link	1.5 Meat, 1 Fat	
		285 Calories	
SNACK	**Nuts n' Fruit**		
4	Walnut halves	1 Fat	
1 medium	Apple	1 Fruit	
		105 calories	
LUNCH	**Spinach & Chicken Pasta Salad**		
½ cup	Whole grain, rice, or quinoa pasta, cooked	1 G&S	Mix everything. Easy and yummy! Splash lemon for your salad.
3 oz.	Chicken breast, cooked or grilled, chopped	3 Meat	
3½ cups	Salad mix/baby spinach	1 NSV	
1 cup	Cherry tomatoes	1 NSV	
		235 calories	
SNACK	**Fruit & Yogurt**		
6 oz.	Nonfat plain Greek yogurt	2 Meat, 0.5 Milk	
⅔ cup	Strawberries	0.5 Fruit	
		145 calories	
DINNER	**Spicy Pork & Salsa**		
1 serving	*Pork Adobo* Serve with:	4 Meat	*See recipe list.*
½ cup	Salsa	1 NSV	
½ cup	Brown rice, steamed	1 G&S	
½ cup	Broccoli, steamed	1 NSV	
		270 calories	
DESSERT	**Affogato**		
¼ cup	Low-fat vanilla ice cream	0.5 Milk, 0.5 Fat	Pour coffee over ice cream and top with whipped cream.
⅛ cup	Extra strong instant coffee	0.5 Sugar Free	
1 Tbsp.	Whipped cream	1 Fat	
		143 calories	

1,400 CALORIE FOOD PLAN: *Day 1*

AMOUNT		FREEBIES	INSTRUCTIONS
BREAKFAST	**Banana Walnut Steel Cut Oatmeal**		
1 serving	*Banana Walnut Steel Cut Oatmeal*	1 G&S, 1 Meat, 1 Fat	*See recipe list.*
2 Tbsp.	Flaxseed meal	1 Fat	Add flaxseed
¾ cup	Blueberries	1 Fruit	meal and blue-
1 cup	Low-fat 1% or nonfat milk	1 Milk	berries to oatmeal
		355 calories	after warming up.
			Serve milk on
			the side.
SNACK	**Cheese & Crackers**		
1½ oz.	Lite creamy cheese	1 Meat, 0.5 Fat	
1 oz.	Whole grain or rice crackers	1 G&S	
		135 calories	
LUNCH	**Turkey Pita Pocket**		
1	Whole grain pita pocket	2 G&S	Stuff pita with
½ cup	Non-starchy mixed vegetables	1 NSV	mixed vegetables,
	such as lettuce, tomato, sprouts,		turkey slices, and
	pepperoncini		avocado. Serve
3 oz.	Turkey deli slices	3 Meat	carrots on the
2 Tbsp.	Avocado	1 Fat	side.
15	Baby carrots	1 NSV	
		360 calories	
SNACK	**Veggie & Hummus Platter**		
1 cup	Celery sticks, baby carrots,	1 NSV	*See recipe list.*
	bell peppers (sliced)		
¼ cup	*Zesty Hummus*	1 G&S, 0.5 Meat,	
		0.5 Fat	
		145 calories	
DINNER	**Fish and Rice**		
1 serving	*Thai Soy Cilantro Fish*	4 Meat, 0.5 Fat	*See recipe list.*
½ cup	Steamed jasmine rice	1 G&S	Spray asparagus
8	Asparagus spears	1 NSV	lightly with olive
1 spray	Oil	Free	oil and roast
		268 calories	alongside fish for
			10 minutes.
DESSERT	**Dark Chocolate & Dried Figs**		
15 grams	Dark chocolate, 70% or more dark	1 Fat, 1 Sugar	
3	Dried figs	1 Fruit	
		165 calories	

1,400 Calorie Food Plan: *Day 2*

AMOUNT		FREEBIES	INSTRUCTIONS
BREAKFAST	Open Face Breakfast a la Med		
1	Whole grain English muffin	1.5 G&S	Toast English muffin, spread one half with cream cheese and layer with salmon, tomato, and spinach. Do the same for the other half of the muffin and have them open-faced. Serve with a glass of milk on the side.
1 Tbsp.	Fat-free cream cheese	Free	
2 oz.	Smoked salmon	2 Meat, 1 Fat	
2	Tomato slices	0.25 NSV	
½ cup	Raw spinach	0.25 NSV	
1 cup	Low-fat 1% or nonfat milk	1 Milk	
		333 calories	
SNACK	Cheese & Crackers		
1 oz.	Low-fat cheese	1 Meat, 0.5 Fat	
1 oz.	Whole grain or rice crackers	1 G&S	
		135 calories	
LUNCH	Egg Salad Tacos		
2	Eggs, hard boiled and chopped	2 Meat, 2 Fat	Mix eggs, mustard, and shallots together, then spread evenly on each tortilla. Sprinkle lettuce evenly on top of the egg mixture and fold. Enjoy an apple on the side.
1 Tbsp.	Dijon mustard	Free	
1 small	Shallot, finely diced (alternative: 2 Tbsp. celery)	1 NSV	
2 leaves	Romaine lettuce	NSV	
2	Corn tortilla 5-inch diameter	2 G&S	
1 medium	Apple	1 Fruit	
		395 calories	
SNACK	Yogurt & Berries		
6 oz.	Nonfat plain Greek yogurt	2 Meat, 0.5 Milk	
¾ cup	Blueberries	1 Fruit	
		175 calories	
DINNER	Spaghetti & Meat Sauce		
½ cup	Whole grain, rice, or quinoa pasta	1 G&S	Cook pasta. Combine browned ground turkey with marinara sauce and heat; pour over pasta and top with Parmesan. Toss green beans in oil and vinegar and enjoy on the side.
½ cup	Low-fat tomato marinara sauce	2 NSV, 0.5 Fat	
2 oz.	Lean ground turkey, browned	2 Meat, 1 Fat	
½ cup	Green beans, steamed	1 NSV	
1 spray	Oil	Free	
½ Tbsp.	Red wine vinegar	Free	
		293 calories	

1,400 CALORIE FOOD PLAN: *Day 3*

AMOUNT		FREEBIES	INSTRUCTIONS
BREAKFAST	**High Fiber Cereal & Nuts**		
½ cup	High fiber cereal	1 G&S	Mix everything
1 cup	Low-fat 1% or nonfat milk	1 Milk	in a bowl. It's that
4	Walnut halves, crushed into small pieces	1 Fat	simple.
1¼ cup	Strawberries, sliced	1 Fruit	
		275 calories	
SNACK	**Egg & Apple**		
1	Hard boiled egg	1 Meat, 1 Fat	
1	Small apple, cut into slices	1 Fruit	
		135 calories	
LUNCH	**Smoked Salmon Tea Sandwiches**		
2 slices	Dark rye bread	2 G&S	Layer everything
2 oz.	Smoked salmon	2 Meat	to make a refresh-
2 Tbsp.	Fat-free cream cheese	Free	ing sandwich.
1 Tbsp.	Capers	Free	You can spread
1 slice	Red onion	0.5 NSV	mustard if you
4 thin slices	Tomato	0.5 NSV	want.
4 thin slices	Cucumber	NSV	
		255 calories	
SNACK	**Pineapple Parfait**		
¼ cup	Cottage cheese, nonfat	1 Meat	Mix everything
¾ cup	Pineapple chunks	1 Fruit	together.
		95 calories	
DINNER	**Paprika Chicken & Roasted Vegetables**		
3 oz.	Chicken breast	3 Meat	Sprinkle lemon
1 Tbsp.	Lemon juice	Free	and paprika on
¼ tsp.	Paprika	Free	both sides of
½ cup	Sweet potatoes, baked	1 G&S	chicken. Wrap 1 sweet potato in
1 serving	*Roasted Vegetables*	2 NSV, 0.5 Fat	foil. Bake both
¾ cup	Blueberries	1 Fruit	items in oven at
		318 calories	375°F for 20–25 minutes. *See recipe list.* Serve blueberries on the side.

1,400 CALORIE FOOD PLAN: *Day 4*

AMOUNT		FREEBIES	INSTRUCTIONS
BREAKFAST	Quinoa-Coconut Wake-up Bowl		
½ cup	Quinoa, cooked	1.5 G&S, 0.5 Meat	Mix everything
½ cup	Mango or fruit of choice, cut up	1 Fruit	together. Enjoy
1 Tbsp.	Shredded coconut, sweetened	1 Fat	glass of milk on
1 cup	Low-fat 1% or nonfat milk	1 Milk	the side.
		333 calories	
SNACK	Veggie & Hummus Platter		
1 cup	Celery sticks, baby carrots, bell peppers (sliced)	1 NSV	*See recipe list.*
¼ cup	*Zesty Hummus*	1 G&S, 0.5 Meat, 0.5 Fat	
		145 calories	
LUNCH	No-Mayo Tuna Salad		
2 oz.	Canned tuna in water	2 Meat	Drain the tuna.
1 cup	Cherry tomatoes	1 NSV	Mix tuna and
½ cup	Beans (canned, cooked, or vacuum packed)	1 G&S	everything else together. Serve
3½ cups	Salad mix/ baby spinach	1 NSV	cantaloupe on the
2 Tbsp.	Avocado	1 Fat	side.
1 Tbsp.	Salad dressing or vinaigrette, light	0.5 Fat	
¾ cup	Cantaloupe or fruit of choice, cubed	1 Fruit	
		328 calories	
SNACK	Yogurt & Berries		
6 oz.	Nonfat plain Greek yogurt	2 Meat, 0.5 Milk	
¾ cup	Blueberries	1 Fruit	
		175 calories	
DINNER	Meatloaf and Veggies		
1 serving	*Heart Healthy Turkey Meatloaf*	3.5 Meat, 1 NSV, 0.5 Fat	*See recipe list.* Toss broccoli with olive oil and
½ cup	Broccoli, steamed	1 NSV	lemon juice and
1 spray	Olive oil	Free	serve on the side
1 Tbsp.	Lemon juice	Free	with cannellini bean puree.
½ cup	*Tuscan White Bean Puree*	1 G&S, 1 Meat, 0.5 Fat	*See recipe list.*
1 cup	Low-fat 1% or nonfat milk	1 Milk	Enjoy milk on the
		423 calories	side.

1,400 CALORIE FOOD PLAN: *Day 5*

AMOUNT		FREEBIES	INSTRUCTIONS
BREAKFAST	Sausage, Egg, & Tomato Sandwich		
2½ oz.	Chicken sausage link	1.5 Meat, 1 Fat	Assemble every-
1	Egg, whole	1 Meat, 1 Fat	thing together
1 slice	Whole grain, rice, or corn toast	1 G&S	and enjoy milk
1 tsp.	Butter (for toast)	1 Fat	on the side.
1	Tomato, quartered	1 NSV	
1 cup	Low-fat 1% or nonfat milk	1 Milk	
		413 calories	
SNACK	Sweet Potato & Greek Yogurt		
6 oz.	Nonfat plain Greek yogurt	2 Meat, 0.5 Milk	Use leftover
½ cup	Sweet potato, baked	1 G&S	sweet potato and
		195 calories	mix with Greek
			yogurt.
LUNCH	Soup & Ham 'n' Cheese Sandwich		
1 cup	Low-fat tomato soup	2 NSV	Heat soup in
	(made with water)		microwave.
2 slices	Whole grain, rice, or corn toast	2 G&S	Layer ham,
2 oz.	Low-fat cheddar cheese	2 Meat, 1 Fat	cheese, and Dijon
1 oz.	Ham, sliced, 99% fat-free	1 Meat	on bread and
1 Tbsp.	Dijon mustard	Free	assemble.
15	Baby carrots	1 NSV	
		380 calories	
SNACK	Nuts 'n' Fruit		
4	Walnut halves	1 Fat	
1 medium	Apple	1 Fruit	
		105 calories	
DINNER	Farro and Shrimp		
1 serving	*Farro Roasted Vegetable Salad*	2 G&S, 2 NSV, 1 Meat, 0.5 Fat	*See recipe list.* For shrimp: put
4	Shrimp, medium, to serve on the side	1 Meat	on two skewers, sprinkle with
1 Tbsp.	Lime juice	Free	lime juice and
		303 calories	grill. Serve on the side.
DESSERT	Dark Chocolate & Dried Apricots		
15 grams	Dark chocolate, 70% or more dark	1 Fat, 1 Sugar	
5	Dried apricot halves	1 Fruit	
		165 calories	

1,400 Calorie Food Plan: *Day 6*

AMOUNT		FREEBIES	INSTRUCTIONS
BREAKFAST	**Morning Smoothie**		
4 oz.	Nonfat plain Greek yogurt	1 Meat, 0.3 Milk	Blend everything
1 cup	Low-fat 1% milk or nonfat milk	1 Milk	together and
½ cup	Cooked oatmeal	1 G&S	enjoy!
	(or ¼ cup uncooked)		
1¼ cup	Strawberries	1 Fruit	
2 Tbsp.	Flaxseed meal, ground	1 Fat	
		338 calories	
SNACK	**Mango Parfait**		
½ cup	Mango or fruit of choice, cut up	1 Fruit	
¼ cup	Cottage cheese, nonfat	1 Meat	
		95 calories	
LUNCH	**Arugula Salmon Salad**		
1 cup	Whole grain, rice, or quinoa pasta	2 G&S	Mix all ingredi-
2 oz.	Canned salmon, water packed,	2 Meat, 1 Fat	ents thoroughly
	drained		in a bowl. Serve
2½ cups	Arugula	1 NSV	cantaloupe on the
½ lemon	Juice from ½ lemon	Fruit	side.
1 spray	Olive oil	Free	
To taste	Dried chili flakes, salt & pepper	Free	
¾ cup	Cantaloupe, cut up	1 Fruit	
		355 calories	
SNACK	**Veggie & Hummus Platter**		
1 cup	Celery sticks, baby carrots,	1 NSV	*See recipe list.*
	bell peppers (sliced)		Serve pineapple
¼ cup	*Zesty Hummus*	1 G&S, 0.5 Meat,	on the side.
		0.5 Fat	
¾ cup	Pineapple, on the side	1 Fruit	
		205 calories	
DINNER	**Mexican Fiesta Night**		
1 serving	*Spicy Steak Fajitas*	3 Meat, 1.5 Fat, 1 NSV,	*See recipe list.*
		1 G&S	
½ serving	*Roasted Vegetables*	1 NSV, 0.25 Fat	*See recipe list.*
¼ cup	Salsa	0.5 NSV	Top fajita with
		393 calories	salsa.

1,400 CALORIE FOOD PLAN: *Day 7*

AMOUNT		FREEBIES	INSTRUCTIONS
BREAKFAST	**French Toast & Strawberries with Sausage**		
2	Egg whites, beaten and combined with 1 Tbsp. water	1 Meat	Combine egg, water, and vanilla and beat. Dip each slice of bread in the egg mixture and fry in a nonstick pan coated lightly with canola oil (use a sprayer). Top with strawberries and syrup. Serve milk and chicken sausage on the side.
1 tsp.	Vanilla extract, added to egg and water	Free	
2 slices	Whole grain, rice, or corn bread	2 G&S	
¾ cup	Strawberries, sliced	0.5 Fruit	
1 Tbsp.	Maple syrup	1 Sugar	
1 spray	Oil	Free	
1 cup	Low-fat 1% or nonfat milk	1 Milk	
2½ oz.	Chicken sausage link	1.5 Meat, 1 Fat	
		473 Calories	
SNACK	**Nuts n' Fruit**		
4	Walnut halves	1 Fat	
1 medium	Apple	1 Fruit	
		105 calories	
LUNCH	**Spinach & Chicken Pasta Salad**		
½ cup	Whole grain, rice, or quinoa pasta, cooked	1 G&S	Mix everything. Easy and yummy! Splash lemon for your salad. Serve watermelon on the side.
2 oz.	Chicken breast, cooked or grilled, chopped	2 Meat	
3½ cups	Salad mix/baby spinach	1 NSV	
1 cup	Cherry tomatoes	1 NSV	
1¼ cup	Watermelon, sliced	1 Fruit	
		260 calories	
SNACK	**Fruit & Yogurt**		
6 oz.	Nonfat plain Greek yogurt	2 Meat, 0.5 Milk	
⅔ cup	Strawberries	0.5 Fruit	
		145 calories	
DINNER	**Spicy Pork & Salsa**		
1 serving	*Pork Adobo* Serve with:	4 Meat	*See recipe list.*
½ cup	Salsa	1 NSV	
½ cup	Brown rice, steamed	1 G&S	
½ cup	Broccoli, steamed	1 NSV	
		270 calories	
DESSERT	**Affogato**		
¼ cup	Low-fat vanilla ice cream	0.5 Milk, 0.5 Fat	Pour coffee over ice cream and top with whipped cream.
⅛ cup	Extra strong instant coffee	0.5 Sugar Free	
1 Tbsp.	Whipped cream	1 Fat	
		143 calories	

1,800 CALORIE FOOD PLAN: *Day 1*

AMOUNT		FREEBIES	INSTRUCTIONS
BREAKFAST	**Banana Walnut Steel Cut Oatmeal**		
1 serving	*Banana Walnut Steel Cut Oatmeal*	1 G&S, 1 Meat, 1 Fat	*See recipe list.*
2 Tbsp.	Flaxseed Meal	1 Fat	Add flaxseed
¾ cup	Blueberries	1 Fruit	meal and blue-
1 cup	Low-fat 1% or nonfat milk	1 Milk	berries to oatmeal
		355 calories	after warming up.
			Serve milk on
			the side.
SNACK	**Cheese & Crackers**		
3 oz.	Lite creamy cheese	2 Meat, 1 Fat	
2 oz.	Whole grain or rice crackers	2 G&S	
		270 calories	
LUNCH	**Turkey Pita Pocket**		
1	Whole grain pita pocket	2 G&S	Stuff turkey,
½ cup	Mixed non-starchy vegetables	1 NSV	vegetables, and
	(lettuce, tomato, sprouts,		avocado into pita.
	pepperoncini)		Enjoy soup and
3 oz.	Turkey deli slices	3 Meat	cantaloupe on the
2 Tbsp.	Avocado	1 Fat	side.
1 cup	Vegetable soup, fat free	1 NSV	
¾ cup	Cantaloupe, cubed	1 Fruit	
		420 calories	
SNACK	**Veggie & Hummus Platter**		
1 cup	Celery sticks, baby carrots,	1 NSV	*See recipe list.*
	bell peppers (sliced)		
¼ cup	*Zesty Hummus*	1 G&S, 0.5 Meat,	
		0.5 Fat	
		145 calories	
DINNER	**Fish and Rice**		
1 serving	*Thai Soy Cilantro Fish*	4 Meat, 0.5 Fat	*See recipe list.*
½ cup	Steamed jasmine rice	1 G&S	Spray asparagus
8	Asparagus spears	1 NSV	lightly with olive
1 spray	Oil	Free	oil and roast
1 cup	Low-fat 1% or nonfat milk	1 Milk	alongside fish for
		358 calories	10 minutes. Serve
			milk on the side.
DESSERT	**Dark Chocolate & Dried Figs**		
15 grams	Dark chocolate, 70% or more dark	1 Fat, 1 Sugar	
3	Dried figs	1 Fruit	
		165 calories	

1,800 CALORIE FOOD PLAN: *Day 2*

AMOUNT		FREEBIES	INSTRUCTIONS
BREAKFAST	Open Face Breakfast a la Med		
1	Whole grain English muffin	1.5 G&S	Toast English muffin, spread one half with cream cheese and layer with salmon, tomato, and spinach. Do the same for the other half. Serve milk and mango on the side.
1½ Tbsp.	Fat-free cream cheese	Free	
3 oz.	Smoked salmon	3 Meat, 1 Fat	
2	Tomato slices	0.25 NSV	
½ cup	Raw spinach	0.25 NSV	
1 cup	Low-fat 1% or nonfat milk	1 Milk	
½ cup	Mango or fruit of choice, cut up	1 Fruit	
		448 calories	
SNACK	Crackers, Turkey, and Fruit		
1 oz.	Whole grain or rice crackers	1 G&S	
2 oz.	Turkey deli slices	2 Meat	
¾ cup	Pineapple chunks	1 Fruit	
		210 calories	
LUNCH	Egg Salad Tacos		
2	Eggs, hard boiled and chopped	2 Meat, 2 Fat	Mix first three ingredients together, spread on tortilla, top with lettuce and roll up.
1 Tbsp.	Dijon mustard	Free	
1 small	Shallot, finely diced (alternative: 2 Tbsp. celery)	1 NSV	
2 leaves	Romaine lettuce	NSV	
2	Corn tortilla 5-inch diameter	2 G&S	
1 medium	Apple	1 Fruit	
		395 calories	
SNACK	Yogurt & Berries		
6 oz.	Nonfat plain Greek yogurt	2 Meat, 0.5 Milk	Mix together and enjoy!
¾ cup	Blueberries	1 Fruit	
½ cup	High fiber cereal	0.5 G&S	
		215 calories	
DINNER	Spaghetti & Meat Sauce		
1 cup	Whole grain, rice, or quinoa pasta	2 G&S	Cook pasta. Combine browned ground turkey with marinara sauce and heat; pour over pasta and top with Parmesan. Toss green beans in oil and vinegar and enjoy on the side.
½ cup	Low-fat tomato marinara sauce	2 NSV	
3 oz.	Lean ground turkey, browned	3 Meat, 1.5 Fat	
2 Tbsp.	Parmesan cheese	1 Meat, 0.5 Fat	
½ cup	Green beans, steamed	1 NSV	
1 tsp.	Olive oil	1 Fat	
½ Tbsp.	Red wine vinegar	Free	
		550 calories	

1,800 CALORIE FOOD PLAN: *Day 3*

AMOUNT		FREEBIES	INSTRUCTIONS
BREAKFAST	High Fiber Cereal & Nuts		
1 cup	High-fiber cereal	2 G&S	Mix everything
1 cup	Low-fat 1% or nonfat milk	1 Milk	in a bowl. It's that
4	Walnut halves, crushed into small pieces	1 Fat	simple. Serve egg on the side.
1¼ cup	Strawberries, sliced	1 Fruit	
1	Hard boiled egg	1 Meat, 1 Fat	
		430 calories	
SNACK	Turkey, Cheese, and Apple		
2 oz.	Deli turkey slices	2 Meat	
1 oz.	Low-fat cheese	1 Meat, 0.5 Fat	
1 Medium	Apple, cut into slices	1 Fruit	
		185 calories	
LUNCH	Smoked Salmon Tea Sandwiches		
2 oz.	Whole grain, rice, or corn bread	2 G&S	Everything would
3 oz.	Smoked salmon	3 Meat	make a refreshing
1½ Tbsp.	Fat-free cream cheese	Free	sandwich. ½ sliced
1 Tbsp.	Capers	Free	apple as a side.
1 slice	Red onion	0.5 NSV	You can spread
2 Tbsp.	Avocado	1 Fat	mustard if you
4 thin slices	Tomato	0.5 NSV	want.
4 thin slices	Cucumber	NSV	
1 cup	Cherry Tomatoes	1 NSV	
		360 calories	
SNACK	Cottage Cheese, Pineapple, and Crackers		
½ cup	Cottage cheese, fat-free	2 Meat	Mix cottage cheese
¾ cup	Pineapple chunks	1 Fruit	and pineapple
1 oz.	Whole grain or rice crackers	1 G&S	together and serve
		210 calories	crackers on the side.
DINNER	Paprika Chicken & Roasted Vegetables		
3 oz.	Chicken breast	3 Meat	*See recipe list.*
1 Tbsp.	Lemon juice	Free	Serve milk and
¼ tsp.	Paprika	Free	watermelon on
½ cup	Sweet potatoes, baked	1 G&S	the side.
1 serving	*Roasted Vegetables*	2 NSV, 0.5 Fat	
1 cup	Low-fat 1% or nonfat milk	1 Milk	
1¼ cup	Watermelon, sliced	1 Fruit	
		373 calories	
DESSERT	DARK CHOCOLATE & DRIED FIGS		
15 Grams	Dark chocolate, 70% or more dark	1 Fat, 1 Sugar	
3	Dried figs	1 Fruit	
		165 calories	

1,800 Calorie Food Plan: *Day 4*

AMOUNT		FREEBIES	INSTRUCTIONS
BREAKFAST	**Quinoa-Coconut Wake-up Bowl**		
1 cup	Quinoa, cooked	3 G&S, 1 Meat	Mix everything
½ cup	Mango or fruit of choice, cut up	1 Fruit	together. Serve
1 Tbsp.	Shredded coconut, sweetened	1 Fat	milk and egg on
1 cup	Low-fat 1% or nonfat milk	1 Milk	the side.
1	Hard boiled egg	1 Meat, 1 Fat	
		545 calories	
SNACK	**Veggie, Fruit & Hummus Platter**		
1 cup	Celery sticks, baby carrots, bell peppers (sliced)	1 NSV	*See recipe list.*
¼ cup	*Zesty Hummus*	1 G&S, 0.5 Meat, 0.5 Fat	
1 Medium	Apple	1 Fruit	
		205 calories	
LUNCH	**No-Mayo Tuna Salad**		
4 oz.	Canned tuna in water	4 Meat	Drain the tuna.
1 cup	Cherry tomatoes	1 NSV	Mix tuna,
½ cup	Beans (canned, cooked, or vacuum packed)	1 G&S, 0.5 Meat	vegetables, beans, and salad dressing
3½ cups	Salad mix/baby spinach	1 NSV	together. Serve
2 Tbsp.	Salad dressing, light, vinaigrette	1 Fat	cantaloupe on
¾ cup	Cantaloupe, cubed	1 Fruit	the side.
		393 calories	
SNACK	**Yogurt & Berries**		
6 oz.	Nonfat plain Greek yogurt	2 Meat, 0.5 Milk	
¾ cup	Blueberries	1 Fruit	
		175 calories	
DINNER	**Meatloaf and Veggies**		
1 serving	*Heart Healthy Turkey Meatloaf*	4 Meat, 1 Fat, 1 NSV	*See recipe list.*
½ cup	Broccoli, steamed	1 NSV	Toss broccoli
1 spray	Olive oil	Free	with olive oil and
1 Tbsp.	Lemon juice	Free	lemon juice and serve on the side
½ cup	*Tuscan White Bean Puree*	1 G&S, 1 Meat, 0.5 Fat	with bread.
1 cup	Low-fat 1% or nonfat milk	1 Milk	*See recipe list.*
1¼ cup	Strawberries, sliced	1 Fruit	Serve milk and
		523 calories	strawberries on the side.

1,800 Calorie Food Plan: *Day 5*

AMOUNT		FREEBIES	INSTRUCTIONS
BREAKFAST	**Sausage, Egg, & Tomato Sandwich**		
2½ oz.	Chicken sausage link	1.5 Meat, 1 Fat	Assemble every-
2	Egg whites, scrambled or hard boiled	1 Meat	thing together.
1 slice	Whole grain, rice, or corn toast	1 G&S	Serve milk and
1 tsp.	Butter (for toast)	1 Fat	blueberries on
1	Tomato, quartered	1 NSV	the side.
1 cup	Low-fat 1% or nonfat milk	1 Milk	
¾ cup	Blueberries	1 Fruit	
		433 calories	
SNACK	**Sweet Potato & Greek Yogurt**		
6 oz.	Nonfat plain Greek yogurt	2 Meat, 0.5 Milk	Use leftover
½ cup	Sweet potato, baked	1 G&S	sweet potato and
		195 calories	mix with Greek
			yogurt.
LUNCH	**Soup & Ham 'n' Cheese Sandwich**		
1 cup	Low-fat tomato soup	2 NSV	Heat soup in
	(canned made with water)		microwave.
2 slices	Whole grain, rice, or corn toast	2 G&S	Layer ham,
2 oz.	Low-fat cheddar cheese	2 Meat, 1 Fat	cheese and Dijon
2 oz.	Ham, sliced, 99% fat free	2 Meat	on bread and
1 Tbsp.	Dijon mustard	Free	assemble. Serve
¾ cup	Blueberries	1 Fruit	blueberries on
		450 calories	the side.
SNACK	**Fruit & Cheese**		
2 oz.	Low-fat cheese	2 Meat, 1 Fat	
1 medium	Apple	1 Fruit	
4	Walnut halves	1 Fat	
		215 calories	
DINNER	**Farro and Shrimp**		
1 serving	*Farro Roasted Vegetable Salad*	1.5 G&S, 1.5 NSV,	*See recipe list.*
		1 Meat, 0.5 Fat	Sauté shrimp in
8	Shrimp, medium, to serve	2 Meat	oil over medium
	on the side		heat on pan.
1 spray	Oil	Free	Sprinkle lime
2	Lime wedges	Free	juice. Serve on
1cup	Low-fat 1% or nonfat milk	1 Milk	the side.
		413 calories	
DESSERT	**Dark Chocolate & Dried Apricots**		
15 grams	Dark chocolate, 70% or more dark	1 Fat, 1 Sugar	
5	Dried apricot halves	1 Fruit	
		165 calories	

1,800 CALORIE FOOD PLAN: *Day 6*

AMOUNT		FREEBIES	INSTRUCTIONS
BREAKFAST	**Morning Smoothie**		
6 oz.	Nonfat plain Greek yogurt	2 Meat, 0.5 Milk	Blend all
½ cup	Low-fat 1% milk or nonfat milk	0.5 Milk	ingredients
½ cup	Cooked oatmeal	1 G&S	together.
	(or ¼ cup uncooked)		
1¼ cup	Strawberries	1 Fruit	
¾ cup	Blueberries	1 Fruit	
2 Tbsp.	Flaxseed meal, ground	1 Fat	
		405 calories	
SNACK	**Mini Pita Sandwich**		
2 oz.	Turkey deli slices	2 Meat	Place turkey slices
½ pocket	Whole grain pita	1 G&S	on pita and roll.
1 cup	Cherry tomatoes	1 NSV	Serve tomato on
		175 calories	the side.
LUNCH	**Arugula Salmon Salad**		
1 cup	Whole grain, rice, or quinoa pasta	2 G&S	Mix all ingredients
4 oz.	Canned salmon, water packed,	4 Meat, 2 Fat	thoroughly in a
	drained		bowl.
2½ cups	Arugula	1 NSV	
½ lemon	Juice from ½ lemon	Fruit	
1 spray	Olive oil	Free	
To taste	Dried chili flakes, salt & pepper	Free	
1 Medium	Apple	1 Fruit	
		640 calories	
SNACK	**Veggie & Hummus Platter**		
1 cup	Celery sticks, baby carrots,	1 NSV	*See recipe list.*
	bell peppers (sliced)		Serve pineapple
¼ cup	*Zesty Hummus*	1 G&S, 0.5 Meat,	on the side.
		0.5 Fat	
¾ cup	Pineapple chunks	1 Fruit	
		205 calories	
DINNER	**Mexican Fiesta Night**		
2 servings	*Spicy Steak Fajitas*	6 Meat, 3 Fat, 2 NSV,	*See recipe list.*
		2 G&S	
			Top fajita with
½ cup	Salsa	1 NSV,	salsa.
		580 calories	

1,800 CALORIE FOOD PLAN: *Day 7*

AMOUNT		FREEBIES	INSTRUCTIONS
BREAKFAST	French Toast & Strawberries with Sausage		
1	Egg, beaten and combined with 1 Tbsp. water	1 Meat, 1 Fat	Combine egg, water and vanilla and beat. Dip each slice of bread in the egg, mixture and fry in a nonstick pan coated lightly with canola oil (use a sprayer). Top with strawberries and syrup. Serve sausage and milk on the side.
1 tsp.	Vanilla extract, added to egg and water	Free	
2 slices	Whole grain, rice, or corn bread	2 G&S	
¾ cup	Strawberries, sliced	0.5 Fruit	
1 Tbsp.	Maple syrup	1 Sugar	
1 spray	Oil	Free	
2½ oz.	Chicken sausage link	1.5 Meat, 1 Fat	
1 cup	Low-fat 1% or nonfat milk	1 Milk	
		513 Calories	
SNACK	Nutty Fruit Yogurt Parfait		
4	Walnut halves	1 Fat	Chop walnuts and mix with blueberries in yogurt.
¾ cup	Blueberries	1 Fruit	
6 oz.	Nonfat plain Greek yogurt	2 Meat, 0.5 Milk	
		220 calories	
LUNCH	Spinach & Chicken Quinoa Salad		
½ cup	Quinoa cooked in water	1.5 G&S, 0.5 Meat	Mix everything. Easy and yummy! Splash lemon for your salad. Serve watermelon on the side.
4 oz.	Chicken breast, cooked or grilled, chopped	4 Meat	
3½ cups	Salad mix/baby spinach	1 NSV	
1 cup	Cherry/grape tomatoes	1 NSV	
1¼ cup	Watermelon, cubed	1 Fruit	
		388 calories	
SNACK	Cottage Cheese with Pineapple		
¾ cup	Pineapple	1 Fruit	Mix together and enjoy.
½ cup	Cottage cheese, fat-free	2 Meat	
		130 calories	
DINNER	Spicy Pork & Salsa		
1 cup	*Pork Adobo* Serve with:	4 Meat	*See recipe list.*
½ cup	Salsa	1 NSV	
1 cup	Brown rice, steamed	2 G&S	
1 cup	Broccoli, steamed	2 NSV	
		375 calories	
DESSERT	Affogato		
¼ cup	Low-fat vanilla ice cream	0.5 Milk, 0.5 Fat	Pour coffee over ice cream and top with whipped cream.
⅛ cup	Extra strong instant coffee	0.5 Sugar Free	
1 Tbsp.	Whipped cream	1 Fat	
		143 calories	

2,100 Calorie Food Plan: *Day 1*

AMOUNT		FREEBIES	INSTRUCTIONS
BREAKFAST	**Banana Walnut Steel Cut Oatmeal**		
2 servings	*Banana Walnut Steel Cut Oatmeal*	2 G&S, 2 Meat, 2 Fat	*See recipe list.*
2 Tbsp.	Flaxseed meal	1 Fat	Add flaxseed
¾ cup	Blueberries	1 Fruit	meal to oatmeal
1 cup	Low-fat 1% or nonfat milk	1 Milk	after warming up.
		515 calories	Serve milk on
			the side.
SNACK	**Cheese & Crackers**		
3 oz.	Lite creamy cheese	2 Meat, 1 Fat	
2 oz.	Whole grain or rice crackers	2 G&S	
		270 calories	
LUNCH	**Turkey Pita Pocket**		
1	Whole grain pita pocket	2 G&S	Stuff turkey,
½ cup	Mixed non-starchy vegetables	1 NSV	vegetables, and
	(lettuce, tomato, sprouts,		avocado into pita.
	pepperoncini)		Enjoy soup and
3	Turkey deli slices	3 Meat	cantaloupe on the
2 Tbsp.	Avocado	1 Fat	side.
1 cup	Vegetable soup, fat-free	1 NSV	
¾ cup	Cantaloupe, cubed	1 Fruit	
		420 calories	
SNACK	**Veggie & Hummus Platter**		
2 cups	Celery sticks, baby carrots,	2 NSV	*See recipe list.*
	bell peppers (sliced)		
½ cup	*Zesty Hummus*	2 G&S, 1 Meat, 1 Fat	
		290 calories	
DINNER	**Fish and Rice**		
1 serving	*Thai Soy Cilantro Fish*	4 Meat, 0.5 Fat	*See recipe list.*
½ cup	Steamed jasmine rice	1 G&S	Spray asparagus
8	Asparagus spears	1 NSV	lightly with olive
1 spray	Oil	Free	oil and roast
1 cup	Low-fat 1% or nonfat milk	1 Milk	alongside fish for
		358 calories	10 minutes. Serve
			milk on the side.
DESSERT	**Dark Chocolate & Dried Figs**		
15 grams	Dark chocolate, 70% or more dark	1 Fat, 1 Sugar	
3	Dried figs	1 Fruit	
		165 calories	

2,100 Calorie Food Plan: *Day 2*

AMOUNT		FREEBIES	INSTRUCTIONS
BREAKFAST	**Open Face Breakfast a la Med**		
1	Whole grain English muffin	1.5 G&S	Toast English muffin, spread one half with cream cheese and layer with salmon, tomato, and spinach. Do the same for the other half. Serve milk and mango on the side.
1½ Tbsp.	Fat-free cream cheese	Free	
3 oz.	Smoked salmon	3 Meat, 1.5 Fat	
2	Tomato slices	0.25 NSV	
½ cup	Raw spinach	0.25 NSV	
1 cup	Low-fat 1% or nonfat milk	1 Milk	
½ cup	Mango or fruit of choice, cut up	1 Fruit	
		448 calories	
SNACK	**Crackers, Turkey, and Fruit**		
1 oz.	Whole grain or rice crackers	1 G&S	Serve on the side.
2 oz.	Turkey deli slices	2 Meat	
¾ cup	Pineapple chunks	1 Fruit	
		210 calories	
LUNCH	**Egg Salad Tacos**		
3	Eggs, hard boiled and chopped	3 Meat, 3 Fat	Mix first three ingredients together, spread on tortilla, top with lettuce and avocado. Serve snap peas and apple on the side.
1 Tbsp.	Dijon mustard	Free	
1 small	Shallot, finely diced (alternative: 2 Tbsp. celery)	1 NSV	
2 leaves	Romaine lettuce	NSV	
2 Tbsp.	Avocado	1 Fat	
2	Corn tortilla 5-inch diameter	2 G&S	
15	Snap pea pods	1 NSV	
1 medium	Apple	1 Fruit	
		540 calories	
SNACK	**Yogurt Parfait**		
6 oz.	Nonfat plain Greek yogurt	2 Meat, 0.5 Milk	Mix everything together.
¾ cup	Blueberries	1 Fruit	
4	Walnut halves, chopped	1 Fat	
		220 calories	
DINNER	**Spaghetti & Meat Sauce**		
1½ cup	Whole grain pasta	3 G&S	Cook pasta. Combine browned ground turkey with marinara sauce and heat; pour over pasta. Toss green beans in oil and vinegar and enjoy on the side.
½ cup	Low fat tomato marinara sauce	2 NSV	
3 oz.	Lean ground turkey, browned	3 Meat	
1 cup	Green beans, steamed	2 NSV	
1 tsp.	Olive oil	1 Fat	
½ Tbsp.	Red wine vinegar	Free	
1 cup	Low-fat 1% or nonfat milk	1 Milk	
		580 calories	

2,100 CALORIE FOOD PLAN: *Day 3*

AMOUNT		FREEBIES	INSTRUCTIONS
BREAKFAST	High Fiber Cereal & Nuts		
1½ cups	High fiber cereal	3 G&S	Mix everything
1½ cups	Low-fat 1% or nonfat milk	1 Milk	in a bowl. It's that
4	Walnut halves, crushed into small pieces	1 Fat	simple. Enjoy a hard boiled egg on the side.
¾ cup	Blueberries	1 Fruit	
1	Hard boiled egg	1 Meat, 1 Fat	
		510 calories	
SNACK	Turkey, Cheese, and Apple		
2 oz.	Deli turkey slices, 99% fat-free	2 Meat	
1 oz.	Low-fat cheese	1 Meat, 0.5 Fat	
1 Medium	Apple, cut into slices	1 Fruit	
		185 calories	
LUNCH	Smoked Salmon Tea Sandwiches		
2 oz.	Whole grain, rice, or corn bread	2 G&S	Layer everything
3 oz.	Smoked salmon	3 Meat	to make a refresh-
1½ Tbsp.	Cream cheese, fat-free	Free	ing sandwich.
1 Tbsp.	Capers	Free	You can spread
1 slice	Red onion	0.5 NSV	mustard if you
2 Tbsp.	Avocado	1 Fat	want.
4 thin slices	Tomato	0.5 NSV	
4 thin slices	Cucumber	NSV	
1 cup	Cherry tomatoes	1 NSV	
		360 calories	
SNACK	Cottage Cheese, Pineapple, and Crackers		
½ cup	Cottage cheese, fat-free	2 Meat	Mix cottage cheese
¾ cup	Pineapple chunks	1 Fruit	and pineapple
15	Baby carrots	1 NSV	together. Serve
		155 calories	carrots on the side.
DINNER	Paprika Chicken & Roasted Vegetables		
4 oz.	Chicken breast	3 Meat	*See recipe list.*
1 Tbsp.	Lemon juice	Free	Serve milk on
¼ tsp.	Paprika	Free	the side.
½ cup	Sweet potatoes, baked	1 G&S	
1 serving	*Roasted Vegetables*	2 NSV, 0.5 Fat	
1 cup	Low-fat 1% or nonfat milk	1 Milk	
		383 calories	
DESSERT	DARK CHOCOLATE & DRIED FIGS		
15 Grams	Dark chocolate, 70% or more dark	1 Fat, 1 Sugar	
3	Dried figs	1 Fruit	
		165 calories	

2,100 Calorie Food Plan: *Day 4*

AMOUNT		FREEBIES	INSTRUCTIONS
BREAKFAST	**Quinoa-Coconut Wake-up Bowl**		
1 cup	Quinoa, cooked	3 G&S, 1 Meat	Mix everything
½ cup	Mango or fruit of choice, cut up	1 Fruit	together. Enjoy
1 Tbsp.	Shredded coconut, sweetened	1 Fat	glass of milk on
1 cup	Low-fat 1% or nonfat milk	1 Milk	the side.
		470 calories	
SNACK	**Veggie & Hummus Platter**		
2 cup	Celery sticks, baby carrots, bell peppers (sliced)	2 NSV	*See recipe list.*
½ cup	*Zesty Hummus*	2 G&S, 1 Meat, 1 Fat	
		290 calories	
LUNCH	**No-Mayo Tuna Salad**		
4 oz.	Canned tuna, water packed	4 Meat	Drain the tuna.
1 cup	Cherry tomatoes	1 NSV	Serve it over the
½ cup	Beans (canned, cooked, or vacuum packed)	1 G&S, 0.5 Meat	bed of salad mix, tomatoes. Sprinkle
3½ cup	Salad mix/baby spinach	1 NSV	beans to add more
2 Tbsp.	Salad dressing, light, vinaigrette	1 Fat	color and mix with
1 cup	Low-fat 1% or nonfat milk	1 Milk	salad dressing.
		423 calories	Serve milk on the side.
SNACK	**Yogurt Parfait**		
6 oz.	Nonfat plain Greek yogurt	2 Meat, 0.5 Milk	
¾ cup	Blueberries	1 Fruit	
½ cup	High fiber cereal	1 G&S	
		255 calories	
DINNER	**Meatloaf and Veggies**		
1 serving	*Heart Healthy Turkey Meatloaf*	4 Meat, 1 Fat, 1 NSV	*See recipe list.*
1 cup	Broccoli, steamed	2 NSV	Toss broccoli
1 spray	Oil	Free	with oil spray and
1 Tbsp.	Lemon juice	Free	lemon juice and serve cannellini
½ cup	*Tuscan White Bean Puree*	1 G&S, 1 Meat, 0.5 Fat	bean puree on
		398 calories	the side. *See recipe list.*

2,100 CALORIE FOOD PLAN: *Day 5*

AMOUNT		FREEBIES	INSTRUCTIONS
BREAKFAST	**Sausage, Egg, & Tomato Sandwich**		
2½ oz.	Chicken sausage link	1.5 Meat, 1 Fat	Assemble every-thing together and enjoy milk on the side.
2	Egg, whole (sunny side up or scrambled)	2 Meat, 2 Fat	
1 slice	Whole grain, rice, or corn toast	1 G&S	
1 tsp.	Butter (for toast)	1 Fat	
1	Tomato, quartered	1 NSV	
1 cup	Low-fat 1% or nonfat milk	1 Milk	
		488 calories	
SNACK	**Sweet Potato & Greek Yogurt**		
6 oz.	Nonfat plain Greek yogurt	2 Meat, 0.5 Milk	Use leftover sweet potato and mix with Greek yogurt.
½ cup	Sweet potato, baked	1 G&S	
		195 calories	
LUNCH	**Soup & Ham 'n' Cheese Sandwich**		
1 cup	Low-fat tomato soup (canned made with water)	2 NSV	Heat soup in microwave. Layer ham, cheese, and Dijon on bread and assemble. Serve blueberries on the side.
2 slices	Whole grain, rice, or corn bread	2 G&S	
2 oz.	Low-fat cheddar cheese	2 Meat, 1 Fat	
2 oz.	Ham, sliced, 99% fat-free	2 Meat	
15	Snap pea pods	1 NSV	
1 Tbsp.	Dijon mustard	Free	
¾ cup	Blueberries	1 Fruit	
		475 calories	
SNACK	**Fruit & Cheese**		
2 oz.	Low-fat cheese	2 Meat, 1 Fat	
1 medium	Apple	1 Fruit	
4	Walnut halves	1 Fat	
		215 calories	
DINNER	**Farro and Shrimp**		
1 serving	*Farro Roasted Vegetable Salad*	1.5 G&S, 1.5 NSV, 1 Meat, 0.5 Fat	*See recipe list.* Sauté shrimp in oil over medium heat on pan. Sprinkle lime juice. Serve milk on the side.
8	Shrimp, medium, to serve on the side	2 Meat	
1 tsp.	Oil	1 Fat	
2	Lime wedges	Free	
1 cup	Low-fat 1% or nonfat milk	1 Milk	
		420 calories	
DESSERT	**Dark Chocolate & Dried Apricots**		
15 grams	Dark chocolate, 70% or more dark	1 Fat, 1 Sugar	
5	Dried apricot halves	1 Fruit	
		165 calories	

2,100 CALORIE FOOD PLAN: *Day 6*

AMOUNT		FREEBIES	INSTRUCTIONS
BREAKFAST	**Morning Smoothie**		
6 oz.	Nonfat plain Greek yogurt	2 Meat, 0.5 Milk	Blend everything
1 cup	Low-fat 1% milk or nonfat milk	1 Milk	together and enjoy
1 cup	Cooked oatmeal	2 G&S	the smoothie.
	(or ¼ cup uncooked)		
1¼ cup	Strawberries	1 Fruit	
¾ cup	Blueberries	1 Fruit	
2 Tbsp.	Flaxseed meal, ground	1 Fat	
		530 calories	
SNACK	**Mini Turkey Sandwich**		
2 oz.	Turkey deli slices	2 Meat	Spread cream
1½ Tbsp.	Fat-free cream cheese	Free	cheese on pita.
½ pocket	Whole grain pita	1 G&S	Layer with turkey
1 cup	Cherry tomatoes	1 NSV	and roll. Enjoy
		175 calories	tomatoes on
			the side.
LUNCH	**Arugula Salmon Salad**		
1 cup	Whole grain, rice, or quinoa pasta	2 G&S	Mix all ingredients
4 oz.	Canned salmon, water packed,	4 Meat, 2 Fat	thoroughly in a
	drained		bowl. Serve mango
2½ cups	Arugula	1 NSV	and yogurt on
1 cup	Cucumbers, chopped	1 NSV	the side.
½ lemon	Juice from ½ lemon	Fruit	
1 spray	Oil	Free	
To taste	Dried chili flakes, salt & pepper	Free	
½ cup	Mango or fruit of choice, cut up	1 Fruit	
6 oz.	Nonfat plain Greek yogurt	2 Meat, 0.5 Milk	
		605 calories	
SNACK	**Veggie & Hummus Platter**		
2 cup	Celery sticks, baby carrots,	2 NSV	*See recipe list.*
	bell peppers (sliced)		
½ cup	*Zesty Hummus*	2 G&S, 1 Meat, 1 Fat	
4	Walnut halves	1 Fat	
		335 calories	
DINNER	**Mexican Fiesta Night**		
2 servings	*Spicy Steak Fajitas*	6 Meat, 3 Fat, 2 NSV,	*See recipe list.*
		2 G&S	
½ cup	Salsa	1 NSV	Top fajita with
½ cup	Low-fat 1% milk or nonfat milk	0.5 Milk	salsa. Serve milk
¾ cup	Pineapple, on the side	1 Fruit	and pineapple
		685 calories	on the side.

2,100 CALORIE FOOD PLAN: *Day 7*

AMOUNT		FREEBIES	INSTRUCTIONS
BREAKFAST	**French Toast & Strawberries with Sausage**		
1	Egg, beaten and combined with 1 Tbsp. water	1 Meat, 1 Fat	Combine egg, water, and vanilla and beat. Dip each slice of bread in the egg mixture and fry in a nonstick pan coated lightly with canola oil (use a sprayer). Top with strawberries and syrup. Serve sausage and milk on the side.
1 tsp.	Vanilla extract, added to egg and water	Free	
2 slices	Whole grain, rice, or corn bread	2 G&S	
¾ cup	Strawberries, sliced	0.5 Fruit	
1 Tbsp.	Maple syrup	1 Sugar	
1 spray	Oil	Free	
2½ oz.	Chicken sausage link	1.5 Meat, 1 Fat	
1 cup	Low-fat 1% or nonfat milk	1 Milk	
		513 Calories	
SNACK	**Nutty Fruit Yogurt Parfait**		
4	Walnut halves	1 Fat	Chop walnuts and mix with blueberries in yogurt.
¾ cup	Blueberries	1 Fruit	
6 oz.	Nonfat plain Greek yogurt	2 Meat, 0.5 Milk	
		220 calories	
LUNCH	**Spinach & Chicken Quinoa Salad**		
½ cup	Quinoa, cooked in water	1.5 G&S, 0.5 Meat	Mix everything. Easy and yummy! Splash lemon for your salad. Serve milk on the side.
4 oz.	Chicken breast, cooked or grilled, chopped	4 Meat	
3½ cups	Salad mix/baby spinach	1 NSV	
1 cup	Cherry tomatoes	1 NSV	
1 cup	Low-fat 1% or nonfat milk	1 Milk	
		418 calories	
SNACK	**Cottage Cheese with Pineapple**		
¾ cup	Pineapple	1 Fruit	
½ cup	Cottage cheese, fat-free	2 Meat	
4	Walnut halves	1 Fat	
		175 calories	
DINNER	**Spicy Pork & Salsa**		
1 cup	*Pork Adobo* Serve with:	4 Meat	*See recipe list.* Serve milk on the side.
½ cup	Salsa	1 NSV	
1 cup	Brown rice, steamed	2 G&S	
1 cup	Broccoli, steamed	2 NSV	
1 cup	Low-fat 1% or nonfat milk	1 Milk	
		465 calories	
DESSERT	**Affogato**		
¼ cup	Low-fat vanilla ice cream	0.5 Milk, 0.5 Fat	Pour coffee over ice cream and top with whipped cream.
⅛ cup	Extra strong instant coffee	0.5 Sugar Free	
1 Tbsp.	Whipped cream	1 Fat	
		143 calories	

Chapter 5

Eating Free at Home

THE MOST IMPORTANT THING TO REMEMBER about eating free at home is that planning and preparing smart meals is something you do for yourself, so it should never be thought of as a chore. These days, many people think cooking healthy food is a hassle—and that thinking has to change. With some straightforward planning, it doesn't have to be a big deal. Part of what I'd like you to take away from this chapter is that I encourage you to do some preparation, but you don't need to be perfect. Unless you have the financial means to hire a chef—which the vast majority of us don't—then you are all you can count on. My goal is to get you to improve your relationship with your kitchen, and maybe even take a basic cooking class if you're so inclined. Eating well is a way to pamper and care for yourself, not a punishment. I want to retrain your brain to recognize the gift you are giving yourself.

Now, when we talk about eating free at home, we can be thinking in terms of a single person, a couple, or a family. The beauty about eating free is that you eat real food, so the entire family is on the same life plan! This isn't like one of those mail-order diets where you order a small, sad, frozen dinner to heat up while everyone else has pot roast. On this plan, your whole family is eating pot roast together. You just have to eat the correct portion and eat it with elegance.

If you're cooking for yourself at home, you can make a large dish of something to last for the week. The best thing about this approach is that you don't have to feel like you're dieting. Many of my clients comment that once they start eating free, their spouses say things like, "I thought you were dieting; why are you eating that pasta or bread?" Once you learn portion control and some smart substitutions, you can eat most of the same foods and still lose weight. When I say "substitutions," I'm not talking about lab-engineered foods like fake cheese. I'm talking about replacing processed white pasta with high-fiber multigrain pasta or replacing regular 15 percent fat ground beef with 4 percent beef or turkey. You'll learn strategies for eating delicious foods at home so you never have to resort to bland diet food or frozen dinners—or worse yet, starving yourself.

I know it may seem silly to have a chapter about eating at home, because presumably, we all do it, but these days, eating out has become the norm for many people. When it comes to weight loss—or your health in general—you can't depend on others to nourish you. Food made outside of the home is outside of your control, and the fact is, most times, those outrageous portions come loaded with salt and fat. The only solution is to start cooking!

> Food made outside of the home is outside of your control, and the fact is, most times, those outrageous portions come loaded with salt and fat. The only solution is to start cooking!

Once you've made the decision to take charge of your own food, it's important to remember that you don't have to be Julia Child every day! Just pack your lunch, bring food to work, snack sensibly, and stop depending on the food industry and restaurants to fuel your life. You don't have to cut eating out completely, and believe me, I really enjoy a great meal out on the town, but I treat it as a special weekend occasion, not an everyday event.

Healthy eating takes effort, so commit to take charge of your diet. Cook larger meals when you are in the kitchen so that you have leftovers to eat for the days ahead. Start going to the farmers' markets in your area, shop locally, and support agriculture in your area. Don't leave your health in someone else's hands by relying on prepared foods as your main source of nutrition. When you do, you just don't know what you're getting!

Clean Up Your Environment

Your home, like your body, is your temple. It should feel like the safest, happiest place for you to be. And I'm not here to tell you not to eat things, but if you feel you can't have a responsible, smart portion of potato chips or cookies, don't have them in your house. Why set yourself up for failure? Keep your home a safe, supportive place where you feel strong and in control. This can be hard for parents with kids who demand junk food, but I advocate buying things only kids tend to like so you're less likely to sneak some of their snacks. I hear the excuse "It's for the kids" a lot, so I say nip that temptation in the bud.

Meal Planning

When I talk about meal planning, I mean planning your recipes for the week: making a shopping list, going to the grocery store, setting aside one or two days a week for food preparation—perhaps one during the week and one on the weekend. This sort of planning saves you time and money and makes it easy to eat free throughout the week. When you make a meal plan, you can select easy recipes that don't require a lot of prep work. After selecting your recipes, make a grocery list. You can buy what you need for the entire week without having to make a return trip to the store for forgotten items. Be sure to check out our shopping lists in Appendix B and sample menus in Chapter 4. The shopping lists have everything you need for the 7-day sample menus.

Reclaim Your Health

When you plan to eat at home, you know the exact ingredients in your meals. While some dishes at popular restaurants may seem healthy, they may contain ingredients you don't know about. In addition, the serving sizes at restaurants can be deceiving. The better route is to prepare meals at home from recipes with ingredients you trust and serving sizes you understand. Always remember that the main goal for restaurants is to make food taste good. That's why they rely so heavily on butter. They'll do whatever it takes to make that food tasty because they want you to come back. That's a primary reason why you need to be so vigilant about what and where you eat.

Your Shopping List

Keeping a shopping list is a huge component of eating free. I like to recommend identifying ten recipes that you can count on day in, day out—maybe a diverse mix of hearty choices like pasta, pork, chicken, and beef. Or, if you don't eat meat, a good balance of proteins, legumes, and such. This is your tried-and-true strategy for staying on course. I am including my top twenty-four favorite, easy, and delicious recipes in Chapter 12, which you are welcome to use as is or adapt to make your own. With this starter set of recipes, you can begin to plan your meals for the week. I recommend starting with about ten recipes you like and recycling them, then adding new ideas every few weeks to build your repertoire.

Remember, you don't have to eat something new every day. Plan snacks the same way: finding staples you love and adding new ones every so often. If you're too worried about adding new ones all the time, it just adds stress and takes time from your busy schedule. So keep it simple on yourself: know what works and vary it every so often.

Food Shopping

Review the seven-day sample menu set, accompanied by a shopping list, so you can start to get into the practice of thinking ahead about what you'll be preparing and shop accordingly. You'll be amazed how this simple bit of planning makes losing weight so much easier and less stressful.

Without healthy food around you, it's impossible to successfully manage your weight. And you can exercise all day every day, but if you don't have healthy food around you, you won't achieve the results you want. Today's the day to make plans for the week ahead; buy some healthy food and treat yourself right!

By planning ahead and cooking or assembling your own meals, you *will* lose weight. Schedule one day a week as your appointment with the grocery store and make it a priority. Without access to the right food it's really easy to fall back on those convenience items, which are usually energy-dense and nutrient-poor. The good news is that you can break the cycle of eating junk by being prepared, and you can reinforce your healthy habits by having good foods around you from which to choose. I know that we're all busy and appointment food shopping may seem like a daunting task, but with a little forethought and commitment, you'll find that it's easier to do than you thought. Plus, my basic shopping lists will assist you in choosing foods that taste good and support your weight-loss goals. Don't forget to stock up on the meal-making basics, as well as those healthy snacks you enjoy.

In addition to thinking about good choices for lunch and dinner, make sure you buy a variety of fiber-packed breakfast foods like oatmeal and other hot cereals, as well as some low-sugar cold cereals. And what about for the workweek ahead? Think about lean and very lean meats, a variety of fruits and vegetables, low-fat yogurt, whole grains, and something in which to pack water—not to mention healthy snacks for you to have at your disposal from nine to five.

Saving Time

You'll find that a little prep work goes a long way during your work-week. For example, cook a larger batch of hot cereal tomorrow so that you can just heat some up for breakfast during the week. Prepack your workweek snack items into portion-sized containers. Clean and cut vegetables, fruits, and herbs so they're easy to throw into salads and add to soups and such. Personally, I love to throw cilantro into everything. You'll find that the simple addition of fresh herbs can turn even the most basic dish into a savory delight. Plus, once you chop your herbs, you can store them in airtight containers so they're ready to use when you need them. Check online for produce storage discs that neutralize ethylene gas so your produce lasts much longer. The discs last up to three months and are very affordable. Saving time helps keep you focused and motivated!

Why Cook When You Can Assemble?

It's great to be a cook, but people assume they have to go gourmet and learn to prepare elaborate meals to be successful, when nothing could be further from the truth. When I talk about eating at home and making your own meals, I don't mean deboning a duck on a Wednesday or making beef bourguignon on a Thursday. Those are special treats for when you entertain, if you so choose. I say, be more of a meal *assembler*. That means you cook one or two days a week and then on the remaining days, you simply assemble meals. What I mean by this is use the basics you cooked once or twice during the week—like beans, rice, root vegetables, and lean meats—to create new meals on the other days. If you make these in larger batches, you'll be amazed how well they extend—and mix with other foods for new creations—over the course of a week. Plus, it's easy to be inventive with simple ingredients. Just think, chicken plus beans and rice equals burritos. Root vegetables pureed in a blender with tomatoes equals pasta sauce. Lentils plus tomatoes and vegetables equals a satisfying Middle Eastern salad. So often, the flavor profile just comes down to some added herbs, a salsa, or some simple spices.

> Be more of a meal *assembler*. That means you cook one or two days a week and then on the remaining days, you simply assemble meals

During the course of your weekend, think about recipes and make extra amounts. I like to cook two kinds of meats and two kinds of grains over the weekend, then I'll use them as a base throughout the week, adding them to dinners, salads, and mixing them with other ingredients to make new options. I'll cook a whole chicken and make roast beef at the same time, and then I mix them up during the week—adding beef with pasta sauce, or adding chicken to garbanzo beans to make it Middle Eastern. If I make a whole chicken, it's going into tacos, salads, sandwiches—you name it. One of my favorite strategies is to roast some chicken breasts on a Sunday for the week and then create a delicious Mexican dish using some of my favorite pantry staples, like canned black beans, brown rice, salsa verde, and tortillas. Put it all together and you have a tasty dish that children love as much as adults. Plus, it's fun to institute a family taco night and start a new tradition.

I use the food options that I made in advance so I can simply assemble my meals for the next few days. The best part is that it only takes me five to ten minutes to assemble a meal that has real meat, hearty grains, and so on. This is a lifestyle approach, not a diet tactic. If you learn how to do this, you'll have a skill for life. Roast vegetables and make casseroles or soups on the weekend—whatever you like—but weekdays should be all about assembly. For lunch, eat leftovers. I am a big fan of crockpots too. Just set up your crockpot in the morning and you have a nice, hot, comforting meal when you get home. Plus, once again, you have leftovers.

This approach also works for breakfast planning. You can set up what you need to add to your oatmeal the night before. Just portion out your berries and nuts and throw them into your oatmeal. This is especially helpful because mornings are hectic, particularly with kids, so set yourself up for success.

Oatmeal is one of my favorite things. I cook it for the week and every morning I get a portion out of my glassware, microwave it, and add blueberries. I use a microwave, but if you don't like that, just cook it on the stovetop, add your fruit, milk, nuts, and flaxseeds and you have a hearty, hot breakfast in five minutes. You'll find my favorite oatmeal recipe in Chapter 12.

I also feel strongly about making it easy on yourself to eat at work, which includes being able to heat up your food. You'll need a quality lunchbox with room for snacks and decent glassware. Forget that disposable fake plastic stuff from the grocery store. You should never microwave in anything but glassware. Bring a proper knife and fork so you can eat with elegance wherever you are.

You may also want to consider taking a cooking class. Not a gourmet deal, but a basic cooking class. Some of my clients are so dependent on eating out, they don't know how to cut an onion, sauté vegetables, or roast a chicken. If this is you, don't feel bad; just educate yourself. There are even how-to videos on YouTube. I always search for unfamiliar cooking techniques and then, in minutes, someone is right there giving me a one-on-one demo, right on my laptop.

Shopping Tips: Things to Know before Heading to the Grocery Store

1. **Never go to the store hungry.** We've all heard this one before, but it's true. Be aware that the worst time to go food shopping is right after work. So always have a snack first, and be sure to bring—and stick to—your shopping list. If you go hungry when you've had a stressful day, you'll grab everything that sounds and looks good, and the food may not make it home because you'll snack on it in the car.

2. **Go to a store where you're familiar and comfortable.** This may sound silly, but some clients decide losing weight means changing over to a new, special store, maybe like an organic market. If you choose to shop at such a place, that's fine; however, it's important to know your store layout. Otherwise, you can be overwhelmed and seduced by all kinds of things you've never tried, and you

may end up buying things that distract you from your weight-loss goals. I go as far as to recommend making an appointment in your book. Learning a little about the grocery store will make you a smarter shopper and a healthier eater. Most major grocery stores are set up similarly. The outer areas contain whole foods—produce, milk/dairy, and meats—while the center holds all of the packaged and processed foods. And most of us walk right into this section first! But we're going to change that pattern. Now, when you enter, I want you to stick to the outer perimeter and know the aisles that contain your healthy options, like rice, legumes, and pastas.

3. **Understand what food labels are really saying.** Most food products contain marketing ploys on the front of the package that are designed to catch your eye. They may claim to be "whole grain" and "trans fat-free," but when you read the ingredients listed on the back of the package, you may find that high-fructose corn syrup is listed as the first ingredient, whole grain flour as the last, and that the food is filled with partially hydrogenated oils. Keep in mind that the first ingredient listed is the one that is most abundant within the product, so if junk precedes quality, this food is not a healthy choice. Also, be aware that partially and fully hydrogenated oils are rich sources of trans fat and that the FDA allows food manufacturers to market a product as being trans fat-free if there is less than 0.5 grams per serving. So if you eat more than one serving, you're consuming unknown amounts of these unhealthy fats.

4. **Beware of fortified foods.** These are foods that have lost nutrients through processing, which manufacturers have "added back"

in order to market the product as nutritious. Remember that no processed food is as complete as a food in its whole state, so try to choose foods that are as minimally processed as possible.

5. **Track the trade-offs.** Many foods claim to be low-fat or low-carb, but please realize that in order to take something out, something else must be added. So a low-fat food may be high in sugar or salt, while a low-carb option is probably high in fat. Food companies want their foods to taste good so that you want to buy them, not because they're truly good for you. It's best to eat whole foods that taste good since they're often naturally nutritionally balanced.

6. **Don't fall into the beverage trap.** There are dozens of fancy, "smart" beverages being marketed to us every day, and most of them are really just sugar, flavorings, and water. Think about all those flavored, enhanced waters, coconut water, and energy drinks. Rather than trying to reach your nutrient goals with these empty-calorie beverages, eat fresh fruits, vegetables, and whole grains, and stick to drinking water for the best nutrition. Water is pretty perfect just as nature made it, so forget about trying to one-up what's already good for you. You'll also be doing the planet a big favor by not contributing more plastic bottles to landfills—or the ocean!

7. **Go to your local farmers' markets.** It's the best place to buy locally grown, seasonal produce while supporting farmers and your community. I really can't recommend this strongly enough.

Chapter 6

Eating Free on the Go

IN THIS CHAPTER, we'll explore ways to eat free when you don't have the luxury of preparing food at home. While it can be challenging to eat on the go, I have a lot of useful strategies for making smart choices in almost any situation.

Dining Out

Whether you're eating Indian, Chinese, French, or some other style of food in a restaurant, eating what you need for weight loss becomes more challenging because you won't likely know what you're getting. We have to remember that the main job of restaurants is to make sure food tastes good. That means they're not likely going to be worried about how much butter or oil they use. In fact, they often use more than a dish calls for simply for added taste. Their priority is never going to be your weight loss, so as a rule, I say don't eat out more than two times per week.

That said, we all like to go out and eat sometimes, myself included. When you do, I advocate savoring it and enjoying it instead of worrying or feeling guilty. Eating free means thinking about your intake in terms of weekly averages, so go ahead and enjoy the occasional meal out. Just use the other days in your week to eat well and mind your freebies. Then, if you want to go out once or twice a week and enjoy some wine or dessert, it's no problem. Your body will average the numbers.

Another way to be successful at eating out is to use my online tool for food record keeping at www.eatingfree.com. I see people succeed tremendously with this kind of tool, and it's been very useful for many of my clients. As you know, most restaurants now offer their menus online. This means you can check out your options in advance, plan what to order, and enter it into your record-keeping tracker in advance. Planning ahead makes all the difference. This way, you can still have fun and treat yourself to a night out.

Another strategy that works well for eating out is to keep it simple. I suggest finding two or three places around your work area and revisit them. Learn their menus and figure out which dishes work well for your goals. If I go to a taqueria, for example, I like to order a burrito with chicken, rice, and black beans. That way, I know exactly what I'm getting. I pick one or two items from the menu that are simply prepared and those become my go-to choices.

If you must eat out more than once or twice a week, you need to be more cautious. I often tell people to eat something before they visit a restaurant. And while you may be thinking that would simply add more calories, you'll find that if you eat something healthy as a snack before, you will make better choices and be less interested in the bread, for example. The whole idea of saving up to eat out and starving yourself all day is hard to manage because of ghrelin production. When you are at a restaurant, start with a salad or soup. What you'll discover is, after that, an appetizer may be more than enough for your main course. Or, you may choose to order a salad and two appetizers. It keeps portions small and often gives you more than enough food to satiate your hunger.

When it comes to knowing what you're eating, I recommend asking what's in various dishes. I went to a Thai restaurant and ordered the spring roll, because it sounded light and fresh. However, I soon discovered that it was deep-fried, which seemed a lot less springlike to me! It's also important to ask for sauces and dressings on the side. This may sound obvious, but you wouldn't believe how many people order these extras on the side and then proceed to pour them all over their meal, using every last drop. It kind of defeats the purpose of getting it on the side in the first place, right? The whole point is that you should use about half of the amount of what most restaurants provide. Waiters may tell you things are lightly dressed, but that is rarely the case. In some restaurants, you can watch how the meals are prepared, and what I've witnessed is astounding. I've observed that, as the chefs finish most dishes, they sprinkle everything with olive oil. I asked why and was told it was to make the food look shiny. Other chefs may throw on a pat of butter to finish a dish. These are unnecessary touches that can derail your weight loss, and they are all too commonly found when eating out. So remember, it's useful to think of eating out as celebratory: I treat it as ordering something exotic and rewarding that I only allow myself once in a while.

Parties

In addition to eating out at restaurants, you may find yourself challenged when it comes to eating free at parties. This isn't only because there may be limited options and ingredients but also because when you are standing and chatting, your fingers do the walking. You'd be amazed how mindlessly we'll grab finger foods and just pop them down one after the other. If you know it's going to be that kind of party, do not depend on the food there for your main meal. Have a light meal first, and go for the socialization. Don't plan to eat your dinner of hors d'oeuvres. If you do find yourself at a buffet-style party where people are grazing, eat something consciously—ideally something with vegetables—and then move yourself physically away from the table.

Weekends

As we all know, it's easy to lose control and break stride on the weekends. On weekdays, we tend to follow more of a routine, and we have regimented time schedules so eating also becomes more regular. However, on the weekends, you need to make sure that eating is a priority. We have to do errands and we sleep in, so I say make your social plans and errands around a structured eating time. You may not have morning plans, but regardless, make sure you eat. Plan ahead if you're eating out. Be aware that weekends are when we make mistakes, and do your best to follow the times that you eat during the weekday.

Business Travel

Business travel can be one of the toughest situations for eating properly because you're moving quickly and perhaps dining with groups of people. That's why it's imperative to plan your snacks and bring them with you. While it's always best to eat real food, I understand the limitations that business travel can cause. Always plan, plan, plan. Whatever your schedule and wherever you are, you must eat breakfast. Most hotels offer a decent, healthy meal and allow you to order yogurt and fruits instead of the standard pastry buffets. When ordering room service or off a restaurant menu, feel free to ask for specific preparations. If you are at an airport and you don't have anything with you, find a healthy option. Never go beyond three to four hours without eating. Most restaurants, including fast-food chains, offer salads and fruit selections. Just remember to eat! Otherwise, you will create a perfect storm for weight gain.

Vacation

I really only have one rule regarding vacation eating, and it's consistent with my whole philosophy. Here it is: Enjoy your vacation. A week or two eating off the plan will not set you back. Eat with elegance and watch your portions. You'll note that many other countries have smart portion sizes, as they don't place the same value on things oversized or supersized like we do in the United States.

Office

I think of most office kitchen counters like a garbage disposal. That's because whatever food is there is there because people don't want it. Your office mates didn't want that extra cake hanging around at home so they brought it to you.

It's also common for a lot of employees to bring in bagels, muffins, and pastries for meetings. When I worked at a larger agency, we had Tuesday morning meetings and we always celebrated birthdays at this time, so people were eating chocolate cake at 8:00 AM. There is always a place and time for those foods, and that was absolutely not it. I actually remember people asking me how to lose weight at those meetings, while they were eating chocolate cake at 8:00 AM. Were they serious? If you know you want a bagel at the Tuesday meeting, plan for it by working it into your weekly eating. Don't be oblivious to your behaviors. When it comes to the foods that people bring in, sit as far away as you can from the snack area. Willpower is really a myth, and with ghrelin working against us, your body can only resist for a little while. If you keep seeing and smelling cookies or some other tempting food, you will eventually break down. However, if you bring your own foods, you can make the conscious decision to choose something else without feeling deprived while others are snacking.

Sweet Tooth Cravings

There's nothing wrong with an occasional sweets craving, but don't confuse your sweets craving with hunger. Finishing with a little something sweet is perfectly fine. Personally, I like a little sweet taste after dinner every night. A few squares of dark chocolate and dried figs works for me. Other people are satisfied by eating some fruit, like berries or some frozen yogurt. If you satiate the feeling in a responsible way, you win the war.

PART THREE:

• • • • • • • •

Rest

Renew
Energize
Sleep
Time for You

Chapter 7

De-Stress to Weigh Less

MANY PEOPLE UNDERSTAND THAT WEIGHT LOSS is about food, but most don't know that stress and rest play a big part in the equation as well. Recent science—and my own research—demonstrate that effective, sustainable weight loss is about a whole balance of factors, including our stress levels. This is so because, as we discussed with food, the body always wants to maintain homeostasis, or the status quo. Our bodies regulate all our functions and react to any extremes, whether they are deprivation or excess. Once this occurs, we've upset the delicate balance that keeps us functioning optimally. Once you upset your equilibrium, your body will react in ways that can hamper your efforts toward weight loss. So in this chapter, we'll talk about all the ways that **REST** (an acronym for *R*enew, *E*nergize, *S*leep, *T*ime for You)—my overarching concept—plays into your weight loss.

Renew

People always ask me what the greatest barriers are for weight loss nowadays. And without fail, I tell them: stress. It's ironic that our society rewards and thrives on a stressful lifestyle. In reality, stress is poisonous and toxic to our well-being, so renewing oneself isn't just a nice idea, it's essential to effective weight loss. In my own research, evaluating my own program (which has an 84 percent success rate of people keeping the weight off), I tracked down the 16 percent who regained the weight to understand what had happened. I am a bit of a perfectionist, and I know my program works, so, ambitiously, I wanted to see a 100 percent success rate with my clients. When I interviewed those who had regained the weight, they all told me it wasn't because they didn't know what to do. It wasn't because they forgot to eat breakfast or follow my principles. It wasn't that they felt deprived. It was that they were super stressed-out. Not all of them regained all the weight; some regained ten to twenty pounds after losing forty to eighty. Only one of my clients gained all the weight back—forty pounds—and that person had endured a difficult year, moving, going through a breakup, and enduring some other personal hardships. In case you think he just forgot or didn't understand, I should point out that he is a brilliant professor at Stanford. His weight gain had nothing to do with a failure to comprehend the program. He was just having to manage more than most people could handle while trying to think about eating free. The others I spoke with just didn't prioritize their lives and didn't practice day-to-day stress management—a problem that almost always leads to weight gain. In my experience, most clients lose the weight. Whether or not they keep it off comes down to stress management. Somehow, stress ends up canceling out everything we have learned along the way.

The common denominator I seem to find with all my clients is the standard complaint: "I am very stressed." Most often, they cite their jobs—in addition to family and relationship pressures—as the cause of their stress. And routinely, I tell them, you have three options. You can keep your stressful job and keep gaining weight, or you can quit your job and take weight loss as a full-time job. Neither of these are realistic options, however, which leaves us with a third choice: You can start eating free and learning how to lose weight while keeping your job. With this option, you'll keep your stability, security, success—plus, you'll be thinner. That's the first step toward applying the principles of *Eating Free*: make the conscious decision to adopt a new way of eating that works around your busy schedule and allows you to remain in control.

In fact, I had one client who had an incredibly successful business that took up all of his time. I jokingly suggested that maybe he ought to quit working in order to focus on losing weight. He came back two weeks later and informed me that he intended to do just that—quit working until he lost the weight. Obviously, most people don't have this luxury, but he was so committed to his weight loss, he took this rather drastic step in order to reach his goal. In four months, he lost sixty pounds. But sure enough, when he returned to work, he gained it all back. The lesson from this story is you must learn to manage your work and your everyday activity in order to successfully lose the weight and keep it off. We have to learn how to eat and control our weight while we work—we have to fit it into the realities of our life.

Let me give you an example of the sort of solutions I recommend when I meet clients with crazy work schedules and demanding lifestyles. A client named Kelly came to me and explained that she was a salesperson whose job required her to drive her car to different client sites. She was making six figures, loving her salary, and loving her powerful position; however, a year later, she was not loving the thirty-pound weight gain that came with the job. She came to me complaining about her stress and saying she didn't know what to do because the job made it impossible (or so she thought) to control her eating habits. On the road, she was surrounded by fast-food chains. When hunger struck, she'd find a convenience store and grab some prepackaged snacks. She had no intention of quitting her job, but she needed to know how to better manage the situation, as she had totally lost control.

The nice thing is that Kelly knew she needed to make an adjustment, and she was ready to change her environment in whatever way she could. At first, it was not easy. She had to think about it, planning and prioritizing her weight loss. After three weeks, this became a new habit that didn't require additional thought. With a little conscious effort on her part, she was able to manipulate her circumstances and regain control over her health and food intake. I asked her to buy an Igloo ice chest with ice packs for the trunk of her car so she'd have it with her on sales calls. Every morning, she took an extra twenty minutes to stock the cooler with vegetables, sandwiches—whatever healthy foods she enjoyed that made sense on her program. This simple change enabled her to avoid fast-food places and also reduced the stress she felt regarding seeking out healthy options. By eating free, she was able to keep her six-figure paycheck and lose forty pounds. Solutions like this seem so simple, but you'd be amazed how many of my clients would rather starve themselves in this scenario or just give in and eat at a drive-through chain.

Another great stress-related example is about Howard, a workaholic CEO who reported that, despite eating healthily and avoiding junk food, he was stressed out of his mind. He was a very powerful person in his position, but he didn't feel self-confident because he weighed 315 pounds. How could someone who ate relatively healthy food end up being 315 pounds? Well, guess what? The answer is stress. This CEO needed deep-breathing exercises and to learn how to become more mindful at eating times. Eating was the last thing on his mind. He said breathing exercises were a silly practice for "yoga people." I told him his body didn't care if he was a CEO or a swami. He needed to take a minute to breathe and think about his eating patterns. So he did.

Stress affects your heart, your immune system, and your brain chemistry. It lowers your dopamine and serotonin levels. It increases your appetite so you end up emotionally eating. (Who can't relate to a late-afternoon doughnut at the office?) Worst of all, stress raises your cortisol, which builds fat around the waistline. Cortisol pulls sugars out of cells to provide fuel so your body can run away from its stressor. Remember the example about fight or flight that applied to our prehistoric ancestors? Today, our bodies still prepare us for flight, but we don't run anywhere; we stay parked in our office chairs and absorb the stress all day long. So that extra glucose doesn't get burned. Instead, it goes to the liver, which stores it as fat around the midsection—the unhealthiest way to gain weight as it can lead to all kinds of diseases down the line, like heart disease, type 2 diabetes, and inflammation conditions, among others. High cortisol levels decrease your metabolism, increase food cravings, and make you moody, because stress raises your sugar levels and then drops them suddenly.

When you're stressed, you can't stop to think about smart shopping and planning for healthy meals. In fact, you view those acts as stressful chores, when in reality they should be welcome activities. This is another important point I tell all my clients. The things I'll ask you to do—like when I suggested Kelly get the cooler—shouldn't be perceived as "work" or "chores," because they are only for you and your well-being. Think of the changes you're going to make as ways to pamper yourself, because in the end, it's you, and no one else, who will benefit from the actions you take.

Something else we need to talk about is the fact that we get stressed-out simply from the act of dieting and restricting ourselves. The act of depriving yourself increases your cortisol levels. Something as simple as cutting out one of your favorite foods will add stress and increase your cortisol levels without you even feeling it. That's why eating free means identifying the foods you love and learning how to eat them responsibly so you never feel deprived or depressed about your food choices.

Just as there are two kinds of hunger, there are two types of stress:

1. **Acute Stress:** This sort of stress lasts mere seconds; it's there, it's intense, and then it's gone. A good example might be when you almost hit another car. Your body clenches up and feels stress, but then it passes as quickly as it came on.

2. **Chronic Stress:** This is the sort of stress that we experience all day every day. From our first waking moments, the news media, the war, the economy, unemployment, a local shooting, the ringing phone, the crying children, the rush-hour traffic, the stack of bills, the surly boss, Facebook updates, e-mails, social media, relationship issues—I get stressed-out just writing that list because our modern-day lives are so very hectic. The point is, every time you run into these things, you secrete cortisol, which makes many of us cortisol junkies, as we're secreting the stuff 24/7. That's a big problem, so we have to undergo cortisol management. Can we fix the news, the economy, and all the rest? No. It's all going to keep coming—and in our digital world, it's even more ubiquitous and more instantaneous. It's modern life, and it's not going away. So let's talk about how to manage it so it doesn't affect you and your eating so much.

How to Manage and Reduce Your Cortisol

As we discussed in Chapter 2, stress affects your brain chemistry by lowering dopamine and serotonin. Even though we can't feel these changes, we need to be aware they're happening. If you don't undergo cortisol management and track your stresses during the day, you'll unintentionally create a reward system mechanism. Why? Because we like to eat. It's a survival mechanism, and it makes us feel good. It's also a primitive defense. We understand now that protein actually helps dopamine formation, which increases alertness and concentration. That's a tool we can use in regulating our chemistry. Remember your parents saying that eggs were brain food? They were right. When we eat carbs from good grains and fruits instead, we increase serotonin, which creates calmness and relaxation.

So knowing what we know, we can create strategies to manage our time and our chemistry. Once you understand your schedule and acknowledge your limitations—like Kelly did with her sales calls on the road—you will regain control of your eating and your ability to lose weight. Some of the strategies we'll introduce may seem obvious, but trust me, these simple changes can make a big difference in your eventual success.

These simple changes include making sure you eat breakfast every day. And if you just wake up and hope you make time for it, guess what—you won't or you'll grab something that's conveniently unhealthy. You need to plan for it. On Sunday, shop for yogurt and fruit or premake some egg white muffin soufflés you can microwave during the week. Taking a proactive stance in your program is critical to your success. And it's not hard; it just requires a little planning and a little extra time. The important thing is not to think of it as a chore; think of it as a luxury you deserve. You may plan to get up thirty minutes earlier, or go to bed thirty minutes earlier. Be strategic about it, the way you would with an important work project, and then commit to your own success. Remember, this isn't a one-time quick solve; it's a set of skills you'll use for life. It's not a sprint; it's a marathon.

One thing that works beautifully to reduce stress—and cortisol—is to take short walks during the day. Even a five- to ten-minute walk works wonders. The walk is not for exercise, it's to clear your head, change the scenery, and focus on breathing. It sounds silly, but that little break can help lower your cortisol, so your stress is lower and you'll have better success with your weight loss. You can also pause and practice taking ten deep breaths. I recommend this to my clients on the suggestion of a psychologist I know, and my clients say that five minutes is magical. I like people to do this at high-stress times—once around 11:00 AM and once between 2:00 to 3:00 PM, as those can be high-stress times in the workday. Schedule two times a day to do simple deep-breathing exercises in sets of ten.

Something else I always tell my clients is that you need to learn to say no. We live in a culture of going, going, going, and sometimes the only way we can refocus and regain control is by refusing to accept added responsibilities. I am not a fan of taking on more than you can handle, personally or professionally. It always ends up being a perfect recipe for disaster. And there are other small strategies we can employ for our greater well-being. If the news puts you on edge, turn it off. I'm not saying you shouldn't ever watch it, but maybe first thing in the morning is not the time. Focus on taking care of yourself and fostering a sense of calm, leaving the media frenzy for later, after your workday. If traffic on the way to work stresses you out and makes it hard to shop in the morning, schedule it on your weekend. Remember, it's not a chore—it's a gift you give yourself on the weekend to make your week more successful.

Another thing to remember is that we all need to adjust our standards. You don't have to be perfect. I understand that many of my clients aim to only eat fresh, organic produce. However, at the same time, they don't have time to prepare their foods. So why not occasionally eat a canned soup? Or a frozen bag of chicken breasts? Or even a frozen prepared meal in an emergency? I know you may not typically choose to eat these processed items, but when you're losing weight, and you know you need to eat, it's better to lower your standards temporarily than to skip a meal. By the way, I'm not saying you should stoop so low as to visit a fast-food joint. Believe me, if it were up to me, I would love to see all my clients shopping for and preparing their every meal, but I understand that's just not realistic.

When you eat frequently throughout the day, you control dopamine and serotonin, which gives you a sense of well-being. So in order to avoid the 3:00 PM doughnut temptation, fuel up throughout the day with the right food (protein and carbs). That way, you are constantly producing dopamine and serotonin, which keep you alert and relaxed, and you're taking a proactive stance in the battle against bad eating. I recommend eating every three to four hours and eating breakfast within the first hour of waking up. I make it a point to eat something sensible every three hours and, miraculously, I never feel that I'm cranky and starving.

Stress Eating

Here's something I wish I could tell every dieter on the planet: Never, ever depend on your willpower. Ignore anyone who tells you to "just be strong"! We are all triggered by stimulus control: smell, sight, sound, and our learned reward pathway mechanism. Our environments are powerful triggers, and we are biologically programmed to respond. You need to know your triggers—even if it means making a list of them. Then you need to do whatever you can to control that environment. So if everyone at your office gathers for a 3:00 PM candy bar at the vending machine, you can't stop them, but at 2:55 PM you can go for a fifteen-minute walk and avoid seeing it, hearing about it, and giving in to it. Take control. Take a walk and use this time to enjoy a snack you love, that you've worked into your program. I have one client whose cubicle was located right next to the communal food table in her office. She knew this was an issue in her steadfastness, so she asked to have her cubicle moved, and the HR Department happily did it. She only needed to verbalize her intention and then take action. Without seeing and smelling the communal food, it was no longer a problem. She put herself first, prioritized herself, spoke out, and made a change. Always remember that you come first. And remember, too, that in order to be successful, weight loss has to be in your top three priorities of actions during your day.

If you can't control yourself and can't limit yourself to twenty chips with your sandwich because you end up eating the whole bag, you can come up with a policy. Something like, "I will have chips when with friends and we share the bag." Or, "I'll have the chips but I'll split the bag into five small Tupperware

> Never, ever depend on your willpower. Ignore anyone who tells you to "just be strong"! We are all triggered by stimulus control: smell, sight, sound, and our learned reward pathway mechanism.

containers, only bringing one per day to work." Being conscious and conscientious about what—and how—you consume is an important tactic in achieving your weight-loss goals. I don't recommend keeping any food at home that triggers you to eat more than the portion suggested. In my house, when my friends come to see me, they complain because they have to prepare something in order to eat something. That's because I don't keep tempting snack foods around—they're simply too easy to grab and inhale.

I also had a client who insisted on purchasing a box of See's Candies every weekend when the grandkids came to visit. She believed it was her way of showing love, or so she told me. But after routinely failing at her weight-loss goals, we took a look at the candy habit and she admitted that the chocolates were really her guilty pleasure, not the kids' at all. Once she came to grips with this fact and told herself the truth, we were able to make a positive change and remove an obvious barrier to her weight-loss success. What we realized was that she didn't even crave the chocolate so much as she used it to calm herself down when the grandkids stressed her out. Once we figured out that she was "treating" herself with chocolate, we were able to modify her eating program so she could better control her stress and remain in charge of her own eating. She stopped buying candy for the grandkids and decided to take them to the park to expend some energy so they'd be less wild in the house.

Now these examples I've just given—the potato chips, the workplace snacking, the candy binges—are fairly common scenarios among my clients. However, there is another category of people called *emotional eaters* or people who have *binge eater disorders*, and this is an issue unto itself. Remember when we talked about people who thought they were sugar addicts, but really, they were just deficient in carbs, which made them crave sugar? I had a client who was simply lacking good nutrition and not eating correctly. He specifically came to me to address a self-diagnosed sugar addiction and emotional eating problem. Once we straightened him out with proper carbs, his problems evaporated. Some people really are emotional eaters—which means they have a coping mechanism developed to deal with some stressor—a reward mechanism that they can't control. But most people I see have diagnosed themselves as emotional eaters when in reality, they are not. They just need to better understand—and feed—their physiology.

Here's how you'll know if you really are an emotional eater. Try ranking your hunger using a scale from 1 to 5 (with 1 being "not hungry" and 5 being "very hungry"). Say you've eaten lunch slowly and consumed proper portions of proteins and grains and then, an hour later, hunger strikes, and you feel like you still want something. Your actual level of hunger may only be 1 out of 5, and yet you find yourself really wanting something. When this happens, I say pay attention to what just happened. Many times, we were just triggered by a phone call, an e-mail, or an interaction with a coworker that stressed us out, and we're looking for a reward. The reward trigger happens very unconsciously, but one client told me that she was at home and fighting with her husband all the time. She would come home from work and an hour later, she would get really hungry and eat—cereal, usually—an hour before her dinner. Once we discussed the fact that she actually wasn't hungry at this time, we figured out that the eating was happening at the same time as the dreaded arrival of her husband.

Taking a little time to be self-reflective and examine your eating patterns will often reveal unconscious triggers that can hamper your weight-loss efforts. However, please note that this book is not going to delve deeply into emotional eating, which is a diagnosable disorder. For most of us, awareness is everything. So what did we do for this woman who was eating her feelings about her toxic relationship problems? I told her to practice what I call *3D*. It's something that works tremendously well, and many of my clients report great success once they employ this simple tactic.

> Taking a little time to be self-reflective and examine your eating patterns will often reveal unconscious triggers that can hamper your weight-loss efforts.

Trigger-Proofing the 3D Way:
Distance, Delay, Distract

This simple exercise can be practiced in the office, the supermarket, pretty much anywhere. As the subtitle says, the goal is to distance yourself, delay your reaction, and create a distraction. And it turned out to be the perfect formula for the woman in the bad relationship. Once we became aware of her emotional trigger, we made a plan that she could follow fairly easily. When she felt the craving to eat cereal, right then, she *distanced* herself from the environment or the food. For her this was as simple as walking into another room or walking outside in her backyard. For others, it may mean leaving the office or just getting away from the food you don't want to consume. Next, as you are distancing yourself, you are *delaying* the onset of eating. And during this time, you can begin self-negotiations. Most of us decide to eat so quickly, we don't have time to really question whether we need and want to consume. By delaying the actual eating, we create space to talk ourselves down by asking questions like, "What will I get out of it?" or "Will I regret this?" Nine times out of ten, my clients tell me they can consciously decide, "I don't need this. I'd rather skip it." And that in turn makes them feel powerful. However, the last "D" may be the most important. It stands for *distraction*. In the case of the woman who ate cereal, I told her it was important that she not to go back to the kitchen, as she still might falter and grab the cereal. Instead we created a policy so that when she applied the 3Ds, she would distance herself, delay her craving, and then distract herself by going online to search for her next vacation. This not only got her mind off the cereal, it also helped her relax before having to face her husband, something she anticipated might be uncomfortable. And this distraction can be whatever helps you escape a bit. Go look at fall fashion trends. Call somebody you enjoy talking to, go for a short bike ride—whatever it takes to remove you from the moment when you're likely going to be weak.

I know that coping strategies like the 3D method can seem easier said than done, but clients of mine report incredible results once they adopt practices that make them think about eating. One of my most inspirational clients is a man named Kevin, who began eating free and lost 185 pounds. Just think about how much weight that is! Growing up, Kevin endured a hard childhood and suffered severe trauma, which he carried into his adult life. I won't go into his personal details here, but he was eating to shut down his feelings and squelch his demons. He was someone who possessed a fair amount of nutritional knowledge but began self-medicating his emotional pain with food. However, he had the good sense to realize he needed help, so he began working with a multidisciplinary team: a therapist, a trainer, and me. When Kevin came to me, I explained that emotional eating is a conditioning, a habit he created and one that we could reverse by changing his brain patterns.

As a basic tool, I taught Kevin the 3Ds and he committed to sending me an e-mail every day to tell me how he was feeling. Sometimes he wrote about his emotions and painful memories. Another time, he texted me from the supermarket, writing, "I bought a box of doughnuts and I'm going to go home and eat them." I knew he meant it, but I also knew that, since he took the time to inform me of his plan and admit his act in writing, there was a chance he'd think better of the temporary gratification and weigh whether he really wanted to derail his own success. Sure enough, an hour later, he said he put the doughnuts down and gave them to the doorman. By sending me the message, he felt some sense of accountability and took responsibility for his actions. Even if he had eaten them, I wouldn't have scolded him. My response would have been,

"What did you learn from that?" and "How did it make you feel?" There is no question he would have felt worse afterward—probably immediately afterward—causing more guilt, and then, at some point thereafter, more doughnuts.

Around the holidays, Kevin wanted to make shortbread cookies and give them out as gifts. I just raised my eyebrows. "You think that's a good idea?" I asked him. "Are you making them to give away, or looking for an excuse to eat rich, buttery, comforting cookies because the holidays are so fraught with painful memories for you?" He acknowledged he wanted the cookies himself. I told him if he wanted to enjoy one, he should go buy one at the best bakery, taste it, savor it, enjoy it, and move on. I told him not to make five batches, because he might end up eating them over the next few weeks and ruin any progress he had made thus far. It worked. He moved on.

Emotional eating creates a vicious cycle. We understand that the pleasure of eating is distracting and creates a reward that lasts a few seconds. But I was able to teach Kevin to distract himself by e-mailing me and taking walks away from tempting environments. And over time, I was able to rewire his conditioning. It's important when learning to distract yourself that you create a positive experience instead of the eating. Just know that creating a life change like this doesn't happen overnight. It took work for Kevin to rewire his brain. But slowly, surely, every time he successfully skipped eating by creating a distraction, he felt proud—an entirely new sensation, and one that he liked. So instead of focusing so much on food, he began to crave that feeling of pride and self-esteem. He was no longer running from his feelings and dwelling in the past, but taking positive steps forward. Once his life was back on track, he got accepted to Columbia University, moved to New York, and started fresh. There's no way those accomplishments would have been possible when he was in the deep, dark cycle of his shame-filled emotional eating. Please understand that we've not cured his childhood trauma or the feelings associated with it, but what he has acquired is successful, learned management and applied control tactics that helped him lose an incredible amount of weight.

So, the point of sharing Kevin's story is, if you practice the 3D technique, it really is possible to rewire your brain. In addition, it's possible to measure your progress by creating something tangible that you can see. I recommend marking a day in your calendar to start applying the 3D practice. Get a calendar and set a day. Then, for every day that passes when you apply the 3D, give yourself a smiley face. On the days you give in, leave the space blank or add a frowning face. You will start seeing that, as time progresses, the number of happy faces increases because you are consciously rewiring your brain. Maybe at the beginning, you'll see three unhappy faces a week. Perhaps two weeks later, there's only one unhappy face. Before you know it, you'll see a whole month with happy faces—and that's how you know it's working. Don't expect happy faces every day when you start. Just become aware of this simple action, and I promise it will make a difference. It's also important to recognize why and when you gave in so you can learn from the experience. Mistakes are powerful. Recognizing them helps you identify your triggers, so you can fix them. I always advise people to accept their mistakes. Don't waste time punishing yourself. Just get right back to your plan. If happy faces are too silly for you, use money. Mark the calendar with a dot and put a quarter or dollar for every good day. If you do it for a few weeks, grab the money and give it to a homeless person or a favorite cause. If you go a few months, buy something for yourself.

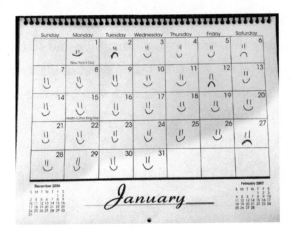

Another powerful story is Andy. He travels for work and stays in many hotels as a result. Every night, he would raid the minibar, eat all the nuts and candy, and drink all the juices and beer. When we discussed this habit, he admitted he felt lonely on the road, but he knew he needed to take action. He was not going to stop traveling for work, so he took the creative step of calling the hotels beforehand and asking them to remove or lock the mini refrigerator. It's a small effort, but taking that action made all the difference. Telling him to ignore the fridge wouldn't work. The reality is you need to identify and remove your triggers. Next, he needed to address his loneliness. He was using food as a companion. Instead, we came up with a list of distractions, from reading books to calling his partner at home. And guess what? He lost eighty pounds because he reshaped his habits.

I believe it's very important to reward yourself when you're succeeding—as long as you don't do it with food. Think about a massage, movies, a manicure, flowers, or a long bubble bath. And say to yourself, *I'm buying these flowers because I earned them.* For guys, I like the idea of buying a tie. I had a client who decided to buy a fancy bike when he lost fifty pounds—such a great way to keep up his new healthy way of life.

So many of us create the "perfect storm" when we are sleep-deprived, hungry, avoiding carbs, and low on dopamine and serotonin. Under these conditions, you are at perfect risk to emotionally overeat. In order to combat the likelihood of stress-induced eating, I recommend you follow the critical principles discussed next.

The Core Principles of Withstanding Stress and Energizing

These are extremely important considering the amount of stress in our modern lifestyle. The same principles that control hunger and help you energize—like eating breakfast—will help you control your dopamine and serotonin.

Be sure to eat a blend of carbohydrates, fiber, and protein for breakfast. It's the most important meal and it drives your entire day. It determines how much you're going to eat at 4:00 PM, and it gets your brain to start with the proper levels of serotonin and dopamine. If you exercise in the morning, maybe have a pre-exercise meal, like half a banana or a string cheese. This will increase your metabolism, help with clear thinking, improve alertness and concentration, enhance memory, and improve cognitive abilities.

Do not skip meals. Because stress affects your dopamine and serotonin levels, eating throughout the day keeps you alert and relaxed. Just remember to combine protein and carbs at each instance for best results.

At every meal or snack, try to combine carbohydrates and proteins. The amounts don't matter so much as the simple act of consciously combining. This way, you get the optimal blend to fight cravings, control hunger, gain energy, simulate fullness, and produce dopamine and serotonin. This way you're less likely to eat emotionally. Protein increases your metabolism and carbs lower ghrelin, which helps with brain function and decreases cravings.

Take brief walks during the day. Even a five- to ten-minute walk works wonders. You can also pause and practice taking ten deep breaths.

Take time to eat: Sit down, relax, and enjoy your meal. This time of relaxation helps to control stress and gives you enough time to send signals to your brain that you are full.

Sleep

Here's what we know about sleep. Contrary to popular opinion, those who sleep the *least* actually weigh the *most*. We assume that more waking hours means burning more calories, but the reality is we need sleep for our bodies to function optimally. Studies are now showing that less sleep leads to increased hunger the next day. Less sleep also increases fat deposits around your waistline. Basically, your body regulates to burn fewer calories if you sleep less. You feel more fatigued and you have less energy, so you have less inclination to care about prepping meals and packing snacks. When you're run-down, everything is laborious and cumbersome. And typically, you will eat out more and make poorer choices because you're simply too tired to think about healthy food. There is a psychological and physical component to hunger. Additionally, when you're sleep-deprived, your ghrelin increases and your leptin (which suppresses your appetite) decreases. So less sleep means you are more vulnerable to hunger pangs and binges.

> Studies are now showing that less sleep leads to increased hunger the next day. Less sleep also increases fat deposits around your waistline.

It is important to note that, when it comes to sleep, everyone is different. Some of us can get away with six hours, while others need nine. It really depends on your age and level of physical exertion. On average, people who slept less than five hours per day were 73 percent more likely to gain weight and become obese. And those with less than six hours of sleep were 27 percent more likely to become obese. With each hour lost, weight gain is greater due to the rising ghrelin and falling leptin associated with sleep deprivation.

In general, when it comes to shedding pounds, you'd be better off sleeping and being rested than killing yourself to get to the gym. I like to suggest people schedule *some* exercise, but prioritize their precious sleep first. We can talk more about that in the next chapter.

Tips for Better Sleep

Start by committing to a certain number of hours (six to eight at least—whatever feels best) per night. Start making a commitment for one to two days a week. If 10:00 PM will be bedtime rather than midnight, be realistic about it. An hour before bedtime, you need to start shutting down and removing stimulants in your environment. Turn off the TV, hang up the phone, get off the computer, log out of Facebook— you get the idea. Then do something to prepare yourself for quality sleep, like reading a book or taking a hot bath. Work yourself up to following this pattern most nights of the week. And remember that you shouldn't have caffeine after lunchtime. Caffeine's effects can last up to ten hours and cause insomnia. Treat yourself to nice pillows, soft sheets, and plush textures. Your bed is your sanctuary, so make it a pleasure to go there.

Time for You

When I talk about Time for You in the REST acronym, what I mean is, time to relax, eat, shop, cook, and all those things that comprise the self-care we just discussed. Don't feel guilty about taking time for yourself and doing what you need to do, because it's the only way to succeed. Honestly, a lot of people fail at reaching their goals because they don't take the time for themselves for healthy living. Weight gain is most often a byproduct of not taking care of oneself. It's not *just* what you eat. It's not *just* that you're not exercising. Self-care is something you will learn to practice and take with you for the rest of your life. For the most part, we only hear about *weight loss* and never *weight maintenance*. And no programs seem to teach the critical time-management skills necessary to succeed. Don't feel guilty about relaxing or having downtime. These are not lazy things; they are essential for optimal balance.

So many people I meet constantly tell themselves, "I need to do more," or punish themselves, deciding it's lazy to sit down to watch TV after work. I remind them that they got up at 6:00 AM, took care of the kids, drove through rush-hour traffic, worked a hectic day, came home to do chores, and cooked for the family. So if you'd rather relax after all that than add stress and guilt about not making it to the gym, I don't think you're lazy; I think you're tired. The idea that you have to be at the gym every day is simply ridiculous. There are other ways—just as important ways—of practicing self-care. We'll look more closely at exercise and how it relates to weight loss in Chapter 10. For now, you just need to know that it's okay to schedule some chill time. Take a nap, read a book, enjoy a bath. Embrace those acts and know that they are as important as going to the gym. Since we know that stress can contribute to weight gain, de-stressing is an important part of our program.

Time Management/Take Time for You

So to recap, what is the biggest barrier you face in losing weight? It's *you*. It's not your job, your spouse, or your schedule. It's not prioritizing and taking care of yourself. And from my experience, I can tell you, self-care is everything. People say their barriers are jobs, bad marriages, travel, peer pressure, scheduling, and more. But usually it's a lack of self-care. And I know it's a lot to ask. We ask you to go to work, take care of your family and your home, exercise, prepare food, relax, socialize, sleep, and manage your weight with record-keeping and meal planning. So how in the world will you do all of it? With smart time-management tools and weekly planning. That means blocking time in your schedule for things you know will help your weight loss, as suggested in the sample below:

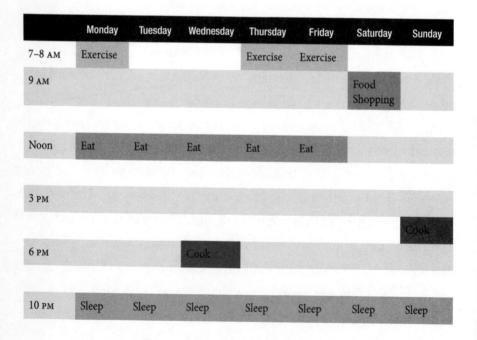

	Monday	Tuesday	Wednesday	Thursday	Friday	Saturday	Sunday
7–8 AM	Exercise			Exercise	Exercise		
9 AM						Food Shopping	
Noon	Eat	Eat	Eat	Eat	Eat		
3 PM							
6 PM			Cook				Cook
10 PM	Sleep	Sleep	Sleep	Sleep	Sleep	Sleep	Sleep

My Favorite Strategies for
Time Management

1. **Put eating in your schedule and work around it as much as you can.**

2. **Schedule time for food shopping and cooking.** Many people tend to go to the market when they have no food, or when they remember, or when they can squeeze it in. I ask you to make an appointment with your supermarket every week and treat it like it's the most important engagement of the week. Without healthy food around, I can assure you, you will fail—so shopping is essential for your success. We'll give you shopping tips and lists later, but now we're just talking time management, so know that shopping is going to be a huge priority. For most people, it seems the weekends are best, both for shopping and for cooking. For busy people, prepping meals and cooking in batches is key. I like to make my batches twice during the week: once on the weekend, and once in the middle of the week. See Chapter 12 for some great recipe ideas that work in batches.

3. **Set up the conditions for good sleep.** Make sure you get enough sleep time. People usually schedule gym time, but not sleep. And believe it or not, sleep is more important. Schedule it and make it consistent. You can schedule your exercise too—that's great. But people who exercise six times a week and don't make time to shop for the right food or sleep enough typically don't lose weight. Once you start managing the time for shopping and sleeping, you're going to see results.

Chapter 8

Not All Weight Loss
Is Created Equal

SO, NOW THAT WE'VE MADE IT THIS FAR, chances are good that you're serious about losing weight. After all, you bought this book and took the time to read this far. If I asked you to rank your readiness to change on a scale from 1 to 10, you might fall between 8 to 10 in readiness. But if I asked you your confidence level, you may, like most people, rank between 4 to 6. For many people I meet, confidence in their abilities to change is low due to past failures. There's a chance that most of you have already lost weight at some stage and then gained it back. That may be why you're reading this book. Past failures affect our confidence in our ability to achieve something now. Our experiences are at the core of our self-esteem, and if you believe you are going to fail, your confidence will plummet.

I don't like to set people up to fail, so let's focus on setting realistic goals. As you lose weight, you are going to have setbacks. That's a fact. You are going to make mistakes, and that is a normal part of the equation. I am giving you permission to make mistakes. You will learn from each setback. Mistakes are a powerful part of how we learn—and they are always educational. Setting realistic goals is part of not setting yourself up to fail.

Find Your Motivation

Before we get into goal setting, let's talk about motivation. There are different ways to lose weight that are driven by factors like gender, age, energy output, and more. Additionally, there are differences in attributes, such as personal drive, experience, and body familiarity. My Eating Free program is based on losing one to three pounds a week. This is not a fad; it is a lifestyle. One thing that commonly slows that weight loss is a lack of motivation. People get bored with it. Diets tell you to vary your calorie deficits. Others tell you to assign a day during which you eat whatever you want—that's all because the creators of those diets recognize that you need motivation. After observing approximately eight to ten people every weekday for many years, I've identified the primary motivators—and barriers—to succeeding with weight loss.

> As you lose weight, you are going to have setbacks. That's a fact. You are going to make mistakes, and that is a normal part of the equation.

Everyone has reasons why they aim to lose weight. It's important to be conscious of what those reasons are. In general, the desire to lose weight is comprised of both a want and a need. Early on, people are motivated because they feel the need to lose weight. Perhaps they feel physically uncomfortable, but they can't always identify their true motivations up front. That's why it's important to take time to assess why you need and want to lose weight. I tell clients to make a list of the reasons why you *need* to lose weight versus why you *want* to lose weight. An example of the difference is that you *need* oxygen, while you *want* a million dollars. When you need something—like oxygen—you'll do anything you can to get it. By creating the lists I've just described, you'll become conscious of your incentives and use them later on in the process of your weight loss. Eight weeks from now, when your motivation is waning, I will ask you to get out the list and remind yourself why you're really doing it.

Different reasons motivate different people: sometimes it's pleasure ("I want to fit into my skinny jeans") and sometimes it's fear ("If I don't lose this weight, I may become diabetic"). You have to decide what's most motivating for you personally. I also recommend being positive when you make this list, phrasing it something like, "Once I lose fifteen pounds, I will fit into that size 8 dress" versus "I can only shop in the fat store."

In my experience, people commonly say, "I'm doing it for my health," which is actually very abstract, so instead, I ask them to detail how their weight creates a negative impact on their lives. As an example of this, consider my client Clara. She told me she wanted to lose weight for her health, but as it turned out, her numbers were perfect. While she was overweight, all of her health stats were as they should be. It turns out she was actually motivated by a common occurrence when she would visit her daughter's school. In many instances, it was suggested that visiting parents sit on the floor. Clara typically found she couldn't get up off the floor because she was uncomfortably overweight. So this scenario was her true motivation—not some abstract idea of "health." Once we named her true incentive, we were better able to create a plan and coping techniques to support her in reaching her goals. I know that avoiding humiliation can be a powerful motivator, and once I learned she experienced these feelings in front of the other parents, we were able to make lists and articulate Clara's strongest reasons for sticking to a program. Another client, Bob, hated that he had to ask for seat belt extensions on airplanes. He found it annoying and embarrassing, and resolved to change his life.

For people who are not exceptionally overweight, you may need to motivate yourself with other things, like fitting into your skinny jeans. Some people depend on external motivators, like a wedding. But that only lasts until the date comes and goes—it's not a permanent motivator. So I suggest looking at the bigger picture and finding an internal motivator, like being able to walk longer distances, climbing stairs without huffing and puffing, and losing that extra fat around your gut that is increasing the likelihood of disease.

Once you have identified your motivators and created your list, keep it with you, in your wallet or purse. You can either read it as a mantra every day or carry it with you for moments when you feel weak and need a positive reminder of why you're doing what you're doing. When you feel down or uninspired, just look at the list!

Set Your Goals

The first thing to know about goal setting is that you should never set weight-loss goals on a week-to-week basis (for example, saying, "By next week, I will have lost three pounds"). Over the years I've had many clients who tried to set goals like three pounds a week. Then, if they lost only a pound, they would become depressed and it would derail their progress. Instead, do not *ever* set weight-loss goals for daily or weekly loss. If you give yourself these kinds of goals, you are setting yourself up for failure and self-

> The first thing to know about goal setting is that you should never set weight-loss goals on a week-to-week basis.

sabotage. You can have an end goal you'd like to work toward, but not something so specific to a day or week. Then, in order to get there, put all the best practices into play: shop for smart food, keep records (more on this in Chapter 9), and integrate fruits and veggies—these are the regular actions you need to take to keep moving forward.

But these actions require their own sets of goals, too. So I'm going to ask you to complete my FreeQ (*F*ood, *R*EST, *E*nergy *E*xpenditure *Q*uotient) questionnaire once a week to understand in which areas you need to improve so you can set measurable goals based on your most challenging areas (we'll go into more detail about the FreeQ in Chapter 11). One not-so-good example of a measurable goal is, "I'm going to eat more fruit." This doesn't work, because you need to recognize that saying it is simply not enough. If you walk past the same fast-food joints every day and only have a vending machine at work, how likely are you to venture out and make a special trip to go hunt down some fruit in the middle of the day? You need to build your goals into your routine with proper preparation. That means you need to add fruit to your shopping list, buy it, cut it up, and have it ready to take with you to work or you'll never succeed. A better goal would be, "This week, I will eat two fruits at least four days of the week during breakfast and my evening snack."

So there are a number of steps that go into setting a simple goal. Saying that you are going to drink less or exercise more doesn't mean anything. Alternatively, being specific about committing to drink only four ounces of wine on Friday or exercising three days this week helps you set benchmarks you can follow. (It sets you up for success instead of failure.) If you do this with a measurable goal, you'll find it attainable because it's specific. Remember, always start low and resist the temptation to set overly high, unrealistic goals.

Set Up a Support System

In addition to identifying your own motivating factors, it's important to identify your support network. Support comes in many different shapes and forms, from enlisting a weight-loss buddy who may wish to do the Eating Free plan with you to finding someone to talk to about your weight loss so you don't feel you're doing it alone. If you do decide to enlist some support, which I heartily recommend, make sure it's someone who helps and inspires you—not someone who wants to compete with you, or who acts like the little devil on your shoulder that convinces you to go ahead and eat that second slice of pizza. Oftentimes, people that we're closest to, like spouses and roommates, can unintentionally sabotage our progress by leading us back into our old habits—especially if they view us as a "partner in crime" when it comes to indulging in unhealthy practices.

Shift Your Perception

Another important aspect to your success is shifting your focus from ways you may have dieted in the past. I want you to focus on the fact that this time you are not on a plan. Instead, you are adopting skills for a lifestyle choice that can comfortably last forever. Making the decision to eat breakfast, embrace your hunger, snack frequently, and plan your food shopping are lifelong behaviors that will serve you well. Your goal is to be eating real food and finding out how to eat what you like in a healthy way. As soon as you think you're on a plan, you'll start thinking about when you can get off the plan. That's setting yourself up to fail. I'm encouraging you to adopt healthy habits, not to deprive yourself. Many feel that because I encourage you to eat what you like, there aren't really any cheating days. That's because in real life, there are no cheating days either. We all have overconsumption days, but you will correct those simply by moving forward and getting on with your improved habits. Thinking about so-called cheating days is really only cheating yourself.

Weigh-In Weekly

For all of us, the best time to weigh ourselves is in the morning. That's the time you'll find your true weight. Always use a calibrated, accurate scale, and do it first thing when you wake up. I like to recommend weighing in one day a week—the same day each week. Not much happens day to day, so checking up once a week will show your true progress. Make sure your scale is on a firm and flat floor. If you do this, you'll see more changes and better accuracy than if you weigh yourself every day. When you weigh every day, you tend not to see the results you expect and you may become discouraged. Worst of all, if you weigh yourself multiple times a day, your weight goes up. Sounds obvious, but you'd be amazed how many people weigh themselves throughout the day and get upset that their weight changes as they consume more. Fluid and food increase the numbers artificially. I had a client named Laura who would always make a 9:00 AM appointment to see me, which I never really noticed until some months into our work together, we needed to change her appointed time. Laura was very unhappy with her new 1:00 PM appointments, and she would come running in at 1:00 PM and demand that I weigh her immediately. Why? Because she was starving herself before her weigh-ins.

Another client named Jeff called and reported he had an emergency. He said Eating Free was making him gain weight. I couldn't believe it. As it turns out, Jeff was weighing himself in the morning—as well as every three hours afterward—and just watching the scale tick up a notch each time. I told him to focus on eating every three hours, not weighing himself every three hours. The moral is, pick one day, be consistent, and don't freak out about it. The weight will come off, but not in the space of a day or a few days. Doing things like Jeff and Laura did will kill your motivation in no time. You're trying to keep yourself motivated, so follow these easy steps and relax. Rest assured that you will lose weight if you do things the right way.

All Weight Loss Is Not Created Equal:
Men

Men like to pretend that emotional eating is the realm of women. But sorry, guys, the truth is we do it, too. Call it distracted eating or whatever you like, but both genders are guilty. Guys, if you are eating emotionally, revisit Chapter 5 to learn about why. For men, losing weight can be straightforward. Some men can simply cut sodas and drop forty pounds as a result. This is because men have more muscle mass than females so they burn more calories at their resting metabolic rate. In this way, nature has favored men.

Men think that when they decide to lose weight, they have to eat lettuce and cut out real food, or eat female caloric levels, which is never the case. I typically ask men to eat more nutritionally dense food. Of course, you can reach your calories quickly if you're eating pizza, beer, and cookies. You can reach 1,800 calories with those foods in no time. But if you watch what you're eating and go with real, whole foods, you'll be amazed at how much volume you can enjoy without feeling deprived.

So men, remember: You don't need to eat like birds to lose weight, you just need to eat wisely. For most of you, weight will accumulate around the waist, so it's not just weight management but *waist* management. Waist fat is visceral fat—the worst kind, as it leads to diabetes, hypertension, high cholesterol, heart disease, and more. For men, following my principles, like eating breakfast and remembering to eat every three to four hours, is more important than cutting way back on calories. Don't relegate yourself to salad—get a burrito with healthy stuff inside instead.

All Weight Loss Is Not Created Equal: Women

For the typical woman, I'm sorry to say nature is not in your favor. You are meant to have fat, and your biology will make sure you do. This is primarily due to the fact that your body was made to bear children. Women can stop drinking soda, stop eating bread, and stop eating chocolate and hardly lose a pound. There are inequities in how we lose weight and what our bodies want. Women have different hormones. Remember ghrelin? It acts differently for women. When you lose weight, your ghrelin spikes. When you exercise, your ghrelin spikes. So the solution, as you'll recall, is to eat every three to four hours and keep that ghrelin at bay.

Managing Menstrual Cycles

Your metabolism increases 10 to 15 percent in the premenstrual (luteal) phase, which is about three days before your cycle starts. Because you are burning more, you experience more hunger. You may already be on restricted calories if you're trying to lose weight and your ghrelin is high, so of course your cravings will be enhanced at this time. Be okay with adding an extra snack. During this phase it's fine to add an extra fruit, plus two to three ounces of meat or vegetarian meat. Don't deny yourself or you'll drive yourself crazy and binge later. Instead, add a little more protein and carbs, and they will decrease the cravings. When the brain is in need of food, it craves sugar—which may explain all those PMS chocolate cravings. Just add an extra small meal, like yogurt and fruit or turkey and crackers, and accept that it's normal to eat a bit more right now. As always, aim to work with your biology instead of fighting it.

Managing Menopause

I can't tell you how many women come in and tell me how healthfully they're eating, how active they are, how well they're doing in general, and yet they gain a pound a year during peri- and actual menopause, which often adds up to ten to fifteen pounds in the midsection. There are a few reasons this happens. On average, women tend to become less active during this time. Metabolism and muscle mass decrease, and hormones change. Of course, your body's hormones have a direct impact on your appetite, metabolism, and fat storage, so weight gain during this time is more likely caused by hormones rather than overeating.

In your younger years, you may have gained in the hips and buttocks, but now you'll notice you gain in your waist, which has to do with low estrogen. So what is the solution? Typically, you'd have to eat less. On average, menopausal women need to eat about 200 fewer calories a day.

If you've already gained weight because of menopause, you can adopt my plan to lose weight. It's just a little more challenging at this time, but if you increase everyday activities like walking, taking the stairs, and things like that, you'll find it much easier to achieve your goals. Doing these kinds of activities is more important than making that spin class two times a week.

If you're approaching menopause and you've not yet gained, start cutting 200 calories a day from what you're used to eating, and that will help you maintain the healthy weight you currently enjoy. Also add weight training to attenuate muscle mass, because muscles break down as we age. Remember that muscle mass drives your metabolism, so if you keep it strong, your body will regulate your weight as an added bonus.

Different Weight-Loss Amounts

There are also differences in how we lose weight depending on how much we need to lose. A common misconception is that someone who needs to lose 10 pounds will drop the weight at the same rate as someone who needs to lose one hundred pounds, which is just not the case.

Losing Sixty-Plus Pounds

If you are in this group, it's always 80 percent nutrition and 20 percent exercise for successful weight loss. The good news is, while you may need to lose a lot of weight, you'll lose it faster than others, often dropping 2 to 3 pounds a week. Remember Kevin? He was 412 pounds at first. He lost 185 pounds altogether. His first 80 to 100 pounds came off mainly by shifting from doughnuts, cinnamon buns, sodas, pizza, and fast foods to oatmeal, healthy sandwiches, hearty soups, and home-cooked meals. Simply changing to healthier foods helped him drop 80 pounds. After two months, Kevin's weight loss stalled and his body needed to adjust to its smaller form. At this point, he was still eating well, but he was eating overly large portions. So, as is common, we needed to make an adjustment by modifying his portion size for his new, lower weight. Once you begin to drop pounds, you have to reassess the amounts you consume.

Say you need to lose sixty to eighty pounds, and you've already lost thirty to forty. That's a lot of weight loss. You've dropped some clothing sizes, everyone's telling you how great you look, and you're enjoying yourself, but you may have hit a behavioral plateau. It's less metabolic at this point and more behavioral, meaning it's a great time to revisit that motivation list I told you about in Chapter 7. It's great to like your new body, but sometimes enjoying it so much—the new attention and such—makes you feel that you're done. Be strong and remind yourself that you have another thirty or forty pounds to go. You can take a break and enjoy yourself, but don't forget your original intention or you'll end up sabotaging your progress.

I notice that females in particular start getting noticed in a way they haven't before, which can make them nervous and self-conscious. If this happens to you, I recommend speaking to an expert. You are coming out of your shell, and there's no more fat to hide behind. Although it sounds strange, you need to face the compliments. This is not a psychological book, but I am referring to a real concern that you'll want to consider. Also, after losing thirty to forty pounds, you need to readjust your caloric intake and do so for every thirty to forty pounds in order to keep losing weight successfully. That's why I recommend starting with a higher caloric prescription, like 1,600 calories a day and then dropping to 1,400. This is because once you lose thirty pounds, you'll need to drop your intake and then drop it again. You may have sixty-plus pounds to lose, but if you start by depriving yourself with 1,200 calories, you'll hit a metabolic plateau.

Losing Thirty Pounds

If you're in this group, the formula is also 80 percent nutrition, 20 percent exercise, and you can expect to lose one to two pounds a week. Just follow my principles and focus on your motivation. You're in the mass majority of people who need to lose weight. Chances are you may have extra weight from stress, due to a recent pregnancy, job requirements, or a new relationship. And while those in the sixty-plus group may also have an emotional component to their extra weight, you are not likely to experience that piece of the equation. If you are in this group, you do need to worry about saboteurs. You will have friends in the same boat as you are, and they will see you making healthy changes and losing weight and may attempt to sabotage your progress. They may be challenged by your success. In most cases, these are drinking buddies and eating buddies—and it's all about them, not you. They know they need to make changes too, but they aren't ready. You may evoke feelings of insecurity on their part, but it's important to remember that these are their feelings, not yours. Oftentimes, it's your spouse, significant other, or best friend. The behavior is not malicious or even conscious. It's really more of a defense mechanism you need to be aware of in your life.

Losing Ten Pounds

If you need to lose ten pounds, I don't refer to it as weight loss. I call it fine-tuning for people who want to go down a dress size. In this case, you'll meet your goal with 90 percent nutrition and 10 percent exercise. This group tends to be comprised of the most active people, but more often than not, they need to slow down and watch their nutrition even more closely. Typical weight loss for this category is going to be one-half to one pound a week. If you reduce calories too much, you will shut down. You are more at risk for eating too little and creating a plateau. When clients tell me they need to lose five pounds, I always ask if they really, *really* want to, because those last pounds are the hardest to come off. You can either stop the wine or stop the dessert, or just live with that five pounds and enjoy your comforts. For you, it may not be what you eat, just the frequency with which you're eating or drinking, your portions, or the composition of your meals.

For example, my client Tracy was eating healthy meals and exercising, but she never gave herself time to eat. She often ate in her car or while walking to work with a sandwich in hand. At nighttime, she would eat standing up because she had to run off to the gym. Believe it or not, she lost five pounds just by sitting down and enjoying her food. It slowed her down, and perhaps caused her to eat less, but in any case, it worked—without even changing her diet.

Losing Weight after Forty

For both genders, this age is the time when every calorie counts. In general, our metabolic rate decreases 5 to 8 percent every decade. And in our forties, we tend to keep eating like we're twenty. We tend not to adjust appropriately. It's imperative that we adjust to our new, slower metabolic rate. That doesn't mean we have to count every pea, but it does mean every calorie counts. Here's an example: if a forty-plus-year-old has a cookie every afternoon (say you do that every weekday), that adds up to three pounds that year—just for that simple cookie habit.

Now let's take a look at some things people may do on a regular basis that they think are no big deal. This chart shows how something that seems insignificant may actually add up to something pretty major. You're not thinking about it, but if you do this on a regular basis, it's cumulative.

Food	Calories/Serving	Frequency Eaten	Pounds Gained Per Year
Movie theater popcorn, medium size	1,200 cal.	10 per year (1 per month)	3½ pounds
Small pick-me-up chocolate (40 cal. per day × 5 days)	200 cal.	45 weeks	2½ pounds
Friday morning doughnuts	300 cal.	40 weeks	3½ pounds
Chocolate chip cookie at meetings	450 cal.	40 weeks	5 pounds
You eat all of these			14½ pounds

Once we're forty, these things add up pretty quickly. Also with this age-group, we have added stress and more responsibilities, so our eating and planning can get lost in the shuffle. We may have kids to take care of, and our physical activity may decrease, so we need to adjust it. It's a time to be more mindful about food, and this plan will teach you the changes you need to make to lose and to maintain your progress.

Chapter 9

Tools to Succeed:
The Success Tracker

NOW THAT YOU'VE LEARNED THE THEORY, it's time to put it into practice. You'll want to start by getting your hands on some basic measuring tools like cups and spoons, as well as a food scale. Now don't let that scare you. You won't be measuring foods for very long; just long enough to learn proper portion sizes and train your eye to recognize what you should be eating when it comes to proteins, carbs, and fats, as well as when pouring alcohol servings.

This chapter is going to help you adopt the philosophy by learning to keep records, which means writing down what you eat and learning how to mix protein, carbohydrates, and fats within the 45–30–25 formula. I've developed an incredible free tool online that helps you track what you're eating in the proper portion size and nutritional mix for your desired weight loss. It may take a little time to learn the tool, but don't worry, it's easy to understand and simple to use. On average, it takes a few days to grasp the idea, but once you learn how to incorporate this important step, you'll be able to eat the foods you enjoy and still lose weight! So be patient and follow the steps. They've helped thousands of people lose weight and keep it off—and they can help you, too!

Your Food Record: The Success Tracker

The online Success Tracker enables you to log what you've eaten in a day so you can see what's left for the rest of the day (for example, if your vegetable intake is low, you could add some to your dinner). There is also a paper Success Tracker format at the end of this chapter that you can use when you're unable to get online. Both tools give you feedback about your intake of macronutrients and teach you how to eat the right mix of foods. The Success Tracker online also includes a weekly summary page that provides averages for the entire week. Many times when people look at their intake one day at a time, they feel discouraged because they may not be doing so well, but once they look at the total weekly average, they realize that it's much easier to moderate intake on a seven-day schedule. The Success Tracker is going to teach you a whole new way to think about what you're eating in weekly increments, which in turn gives you much more freedom to eat what you love. You'll learn that one day won't derail your weight loss as long as you return to your normal schedule the next day. So you can repair one day's errors by simply getting back on track the next day.

It's important to remember that I don't expect perfection. If you haven't adhered spot-on with the 45–30–25 formula by the end of the week, that's okay. It should be used as a general guideline. As long as you come in plus or minus 2 percent of those numbers at any time, and you're still in the good zone, you should still lose weight. The same is true with your freebies. If you are allowed five freebies of grains and one day you eat seven, it's no big deal. The next day, eat one less grain and your body will balance itself out. You can look at your plan as five freebies per day or thirty-five per week—either approach will work for you.

Record Keeping

One of the keys to your success is record keeping because it helps you see where you're spending your freebies each day, as well as throughout the week. So if you consume more than the recommended amount of freebies one day, just check out your summary page to see how you're doing on average for the week. You can use this information to plan ahead for days that you know you'll go over your caloric prescription, like at holiday parties and during family gatherings.

Keeping track of the foods you eat will also clue you in to what kinds of foods you should be choosing for the remainder of the day or the week, and which ones you should probably skip for now. Just having this knowledge will motivate you to stay on the right track.

Your attitude toward record keeping is very important to your success. It shouldn't be seen as a chore or a painful thing to do. Taking the time to do the record keeping is time for you. It's an investment in your weight loss. If there is a magic answer to weight loss, this is it. It's very straightforward. You do the record keeping, you lose weight. If you do half-assed record keeping, you will have half-assed weight loss. If you do it, you'll lose it. It's really that simple.

> Your attitude toward record keeping is very important to your success. It shouldn't be seen as a chore or a painful thing to do. Taking the time to do the record keeping is time for you. It's an investment in your weight loss.

I practiced record keeping myself for ten months because I wanted to experience the process, assess the time commitment, and really get what my clients would be doing. Even knowing everything I know, I learned so much about myself and my options, choices, habits, and behaviors through this exercise. It made me rethink everything I ate, and it was an incredible learning experience. Even with all the nutrition and behavioral knowledge I possess, I am still learning.

When to Record Keep

Daily record keeping is the best way to see if you're meeting your goals and staying within your recommendations. Be accurate and complete with your entries for the best information and results. Remember, inaccurate or incomplete entries are your enemy, as they don't provide a clear picture of where you are right now. Be good to yourself by being honest with yourself!

If you find that you can't keep records online as you go because you're not in front of a computer, my recommendation, and what appears to work best for most people, is to allocate two times a day to do record keeping and make that your routine. Maybe try tracking your progress once after lunch and once after dinner. Don't worry if you miss a day. Just start a new day and move forward! Some people record keep as soon as they eat something. That doesn't work for everyone. The other way you can do it is to wait until the end of the day, but I find that people tend to forget what they've eaten by that time, unless they wrote it down somewhere. Trust me, it's easier to just do it twice, and once you're used to it, you'll do it in no time.

If you miss a day of record keeping, forget about it and keep going the next day. Don't punish yourself; just get back on track. It's very important to see each mealtime in terms of the meal itself, the times you ate, your mood before eating, who you were with, and really, the whole picture of your behaviors. You need to see the three- to four-hour breaks between meals and, most important, identify what triggers you to eat. We also have a way to keep track of your hunger level. All of this will tell you so much about your options and why you're doing what you're doing. Remember, we're not just tracking calories here, we're looking into behaviors.

Truly, you can eat whatever you want. You just need to write it down! We don't want you to have to give up doing fun things just because you're trying to lose weight. That's why Eating Free lets you eat at restaurants, enjoy a night out with friends, and let loose on vacation. Whatever you want to do, just keep track of what you eat and remember the basics.

Using the Tool in Advance of Eating

I have some clients who use the Success Tracker as a proactive tool. They'll look at what they've eaten for the day and use the tool to plan—and commit to—what they'll eat for their next meal. I recall one client in particular who came into my office on Tuesday feeling nervous because he had plans to eat pizza and beer on Saturday. I told him to go ahead and enter on Tuesday what he'd like to eat on Saturday. He entered two slices of pizza and three beers. Then he ate accordingly on the days leading up to Saturday and still managed to lose three pounds. There should be no concept of cheating. You need to manage your food throughout the week because it's a lifestyle approach. And the only way to manage that is by record keeping and really paying attention to your numbers.

The Success Tracker for iPhone App

I've also created an iPhone version of the Success Tracker for when you're on the go. It's important to know that it's a companion, not a replacement tool, but it will make it easier to stay on top of what you're eating and when. Once you're comfortable with the notion of your freebies, you can just enter the freebies on the spot and the app will update your record online. The app also allows you to take pictures of your meal if you can't take the time to enter ingredients and portion sizes. Say you're at an Italian restaurant, for example. Just take a picture of your spaghetti with meatballs, and later you'll be able to guesstimate the portion size because you'll be versed in what different amounts of food look like.

Also, you'll see that in our online "pantry"—the archive that lists food choices in a drop-down menu—we've provided more than 3,500 foods from all ethnicities and brands and their nutritional value. Of course, you can enter new foods or dishes as well, but you'll be amazed at how many items we've already put into the system for you. Just tell the tracker what you're eating and in what amount, and we've done the calculations for you. Say you're eating Chinese food, like Kung Pao chicken. Don't worry that we don't know what restaurant it is because the food tracker works on averages and we've given a solid estimate of likely calories, fat, and carbs. It won't be exact, but it will give you a really good indication of where you fall. We even have a label calculator, so if we don't have your brand, you can enter the ingredients and we'll calculate it. You can enter your favorite recipes, and we'll calculate that too.

What If I Overindulged?

Because your body works on a weekly average—not daily—your weight will not change due to one day of overeating. So if you do stray from your program, follow these simple steps to get back on track.

1. Go back to your normal, healthy eating plan and start recording your foods again so you can easily get back on track.
2. You do not need to undereat the next day. If you undereat, it may backfire by causing you to overeat later due to hunger.

Ready to Get Started?

As you explore the Success Tracker online, you'll see that there are a number of educational tools to help you use it with ease. There are guidelines, videos, FAQs, and more available resources. There are also registered dietitians available to speak with if you have specific dietary needs due to, say, diabetes or digestive health issues. The Success Tracker is designed to be a thorough tool you can rely on as you build your Eating Free plan.

Of course, learning a new tool is always a challenge. Once you learn to navigate it, it'll be second nature. But take the time and expect to use it for a few days to get used to it. Then, once you're accustomed to it, you'll find it won't take more than three minutes per meal entry. For those who would like to use a paper format for record keeping, I've included the format that follows, which can be used on a daily basis.

> Because your body works on a weekly average—not daily—your weight will not change due to one day of overeating.

Food Record							
ITEM	G&S	FRUIT	MILK	NSV	MEAT	FAT	SUGAR
My daily freebies for 1,400 calories	5	3	2	5	9	5	
Food eaten							
½ cup oatmeal	1						
¾ cup blueberries		1					
1 oz. low-fat cheese					1	0.5	
1 small apple		1					
Turkey sandwich	2			1	3		
1 chocolate chip cookie	2					4	2
Totals:							

PART FOUR:

• • • • • • • •

Energy Expenditures

Chapter 10

How Working Out Can Derail Your Weight Loss

WHEN MOST PEOPLE THINK OF ENERGY EXPENDITURES, they think only of exercise. But in reality, there are three important components that will determine your calorie expenditures for the day, or your total energy expenditure (TEE). The first component is your resting metabolic rate, which means your metabolism as it was described in Chapter 2. Your resting metabolic rate represents the calories the body burns to maintain vital body functions (heart rate, brain function, breathing, etc.). In simple terms, it is the number of calories you would burn if you were awake, but at rest all day with no physical exertion.

The second component that determines your energy expenditure is the amount of activity you do during the day through your work. Depending upon the activity level you perform during the day, your calories burned will vary. Even a sedentary person who sits in front of a computer will burn a small number of calories.

The third component is exercise. Your TEE is the sum of these three components, the total calories you burn in a 24-hour period. So if you eat the same number of calories as your TEE calculation, you will maintain your weight; if you eat more than your TEE calculation, you will gain weight; and if you eat less than your TEE, you will lose weight. It sounds simple, but it's a very powerful formula to understand. To see an average TEE based on gender, age, and activity levels, please refer to Appendix A. Or, better yet, to calculate your actual TEE, visit the free online tool at www.eatingfree.com and sign up for a free account.

In this chapter, we're going to explore a concept related to exercise that I call the 80/20 Rule. It's the idea that your weight-loss effort should be 80 percent nutrition plus self-care and 20 percent exercise—probably the reverse of what we've always assumed. Like so many other health professionals, I used to counsel people to use exercise as a major part of their weight-loss program. But then I found out that many people were exercising as much as the most ambitious government recommendations (ninety minutes most days of the week) and not getting anywhere with their weight loss. I also kept hearing from new clients how much they were exercising and how nothing was happening. So then I decided to really look into the research and closely study my clients' food and exercise records.

> Your weight-loss effort should be 80 percent nutrition plus self-care and 20 percent exercise—probably the reverse of what we've always assumed.

As I analyzed the research from my clientele over the years, I began to see a trend: exercise wasn't doing what we all assumed it was supposed to do. There are a number of reasons why this was so—things like self-rewarding, compensation, metabolism shutdown, and of course, ghrelin spikes—but we'll get to each of these in a moment. The thing that struck me was that after years of hypothesizing about the ineffectiveness of exercise in weight loss, major studies began appearing that revealed the same findings. Headlines in publications like *Time* began announcing what I'd been documenting for years: for the majority of people, exercise is not going to make you lose weight. You're going to find that this chapter is one of the most enlightening and surprising, so pay close attention. I'm going to revise your whole outlook about how best to shed those pounds. And it has little to do with breaking a sweat.

In the 1930s, doctors used to prescribe bed rest for weight loss. Oh, how times have changed. These days, exercise has been dramatized and monetized. According to the Minnesota Heart Survey from 1980, 47 percent of respondents said they exercised regularly. In 2000, that number went up to 57 percent. That seems like a good thing, except that in the same period of time, the obesity rates doubled among adults—from 15 percent to 30 percent. When you see numbers like that, something's not adding up.

While I'm a fierce advocate of exercise for health (I exercise four or five times a week for my health and I love it), I know for a fact that it's not the primary means for losing weight. So stop working out in order to shed pounds, to punish yourself for being fat, or to give yourself permission to eat junk! None of these motivations will deliver the results you desire.

The question you may be asking at this point is, "How many calories should I burn?" You may be shocked to hear this, but when it comes to losing weight, exercise is not the ticket. I know it sounds crazy, but think about it. Have you ever worked and worked and worked at exercise and not seen the results you wanted? Do you find yourself getting hungry after exercise and end up eating more—either as a reward or just because you are hungrier? Is it possible that exercise is keeping you from losing weight? For most people the answer is yes.

Maybe you've been killing yourself on the treadmill, signing up for boot camps, or even running marathons without losing your extra weight. The reality for so many of us is that we exercise endlessly and never see the results we want. So if you are using exercise as your primary means of losing weight, you're wasting your time. Yep, I said it. Exercise is really neither here nor there when it comes to weight loss. Can it help? Yes. It certainly won't hurt. But is it the means of attaining your goal? No, it is not. I know your trainer, your TV, and even your government will tell you otherwise, but hear me out. As an authority on the subject, I've been helping clients practice proper nutrition and self-care for sixteen years, and my research and observations demonstrate that *it is your overall effort toward nutrition—not exercise—that is critical to your success in weight loss.*

The first thing to know is that exercise is extremely important. It's important for promoting heart health, managing stress, boosting hormones, maintaining lean muscle mass, and enhancing mental health and cognitive abilities. Exercise has a great many benefits that cannot be underestimated, but it is not, I repeat *not*, the primary tool you're going to use to lose weight. In fact, many of my clients become disillusioned and fail at their weight-loss attempts because they threw themselves into intensive workouts that didn't produce the results they wanted, so they gave up. That's because they didn't understand the science of what was happening in their bodies. So let's back up a minute and examine why we think exercise is everything.

> Exercise has a great many benefits that cannot be underestimated, but it is not, I repeat not, the primary tool you're going to use to lose weight.

I'm betting you've seen infomercials where fitness gurus claim to help you burn that fat away in ten or fifteen days. Maybe you've studied the buffed physiques of those "hard bodies" who live at the gym. Perhaps you've watched shows like *The Biggest Loser* that feature scenes of overweight contestants sweating and grunting and crawling through intense fitness regimens in sweat suits so they will shed pounds. Today's media—particularly marketing shows and infomercials—make a killing on programs featuring beautiful women doing slow, repetitive movement, like, for example, hula hooping. I hate to break it to you, but gyrating your hips won't shake off your fat. You could conceivably strengthen that muscle group, and if you do it enough, you may improve your cardio fitness, but the fat will still be there on top of your new muscle. What you don't see in most of the televised "fitness" programming is the nutritional story behind the imagery.

In all my years of working in nutrition, the weight-loss myth I encounter more than any other is that people believe the minute they start exercising, they'll start losing weight. And when I ask clients how much time they think they should invest in exercising, they often cite high-level goals. When I ask how much time and energy they devote to nutrition—to planning and cooking meals and recording what they eat—they look at me like I'm crazy. But here's the reality: learning about and planning what to eat takes a little commitment. That's why I'm advocating 80 percent of your effort be nutrition-based and self-care and only 20 percent come from exercise. For many of you, that will sound like the reverse of what you've always been told. But after sixteen years of helping clients lose weight and keep it off, I have the evidence that it's true.

Interestingly, the expert organizations in the field are finally catching up and publishing position papers about what I've been saying all along. *Time* magazine's August 2009 cover was emblazoned with the headline, "The Myth About Exercise." The explanation read, "Of course it's good for you, but it won't make you lose weight." In April 2010, the *New York Times* printed an article titled "Weighing the Evidence on Exercise." At the European Congress on Obesity a month later, researchers presented conclusions that, over the last thirty years, weight gain in the United States can be attributed almost entirely to caloric intake, as opposed to lack of physical activity.

The big revelation that's come to light recently is that exercise has little effect on weight loss. It has its place, which is to *maintain your weight loss* after you've achieved it. And believe me, I think it's great to integrate exercise while losing weight to set up a behavior you're going to need to practice for maintenance. The problem is that most people who want to lose weight end up killing themselves by exercising as much as possible.

Today research is showing that ghrelin spikes when we exercise, so in some cases, too much exercise can hinder weight loss. Ghrelin spikes in females when they exercise, even if they don't lose weight, and then it increases when they do lose weight. It also increases in males as they lose weight and lose muscle mass, which makes it doubly difficult to control.

Calorie counting can make you lose muscle mass because people worry more about the number of calories and not where they come from. (Most people who overexercise are also losing muscle mass, as they are not eating enough of the right foods.) That's why my 45–30–25 formula for nutrition is so important for *quality weight loss*. It offers plenty of protein and keeps muscle mass in check. What people need to remember is that exercise increases our hunger and spikes our ghrelin. So I always tell my clients, if you only have a little extra time in the week, you're better off spending it shopping and preparing quality foods than breaking your back to squeeze in gym time.

The Compensation Trap

There is also the issue of what we call *compensation*, which is both a psychological and physiological effect that happens in a few ways. Physiologically, when you exercise and lose weight and eat too little, your body will compensate by slowing your metabolism to hold on to fat because you're doing something it considers extreme. When you exercise, you break your equilibrium. And because your body wants to maintain homeostasis, your metabolism slows down. Psychologically, your reward mechanism kicks in and makes you believe that because you just exercised, you deserve a reward, like, say, a muffin. We also compensate by thinking that since we've already exercised, we don't need to move for the rest of the day, and we've earned some sort of treat. Of course, it's possible to exercise and then fight your cravings, but that just sets up a hurdle that many of us end up stumbling over.

Think of it this way: To burn 500 calories at the gym takes an hour of time and a really intense workout, but that 500 calories can be replenished in three minutes when you eat, say, a muffin. So the thought that working out for an hour and a half three times a week gives you the "credit" to eat treats is incorrect—you've really only earned an extra muffin and a half (that's for the *whole week*, mind you, not for the day!). However, many of us use a good week of workouts as permission to indulge in something far more decadent than that.

Have you ever gone to the gym and rewarded yourself with a slice of pizza or a brownie afterward? Well, there goes your workout. That's just another example of *compensation*. Or maybe you work out like a fiend for sixty to ninety minutes some days only to sit around for the rest of the day, which brings your metabolism to a screeching halt. Did you know it's actually best to keep your metabolism going by remaining active throughout the day just by standing, walking to and from work, or taking the stairs? As you know, your metabolism is in constant aim of homeostasis. Little food (energy in) combined with lots of exercise (energy out) causes your metabolism to slow in its efforts to efficiently make use of the energy imbalance.

Although the laws of thermodynamics claim that more energy out and less energy in leads to a deficit (or weight loss), the human body and psyche are determined by survival and pleasure. Hence, we end up eating both to replenish our energy and to reward ourselves for hard work. As we determine an appropriate deficit, we need to find a safe sweet spot. People get overzealous about cutting calories, and instead of dropping, say, 500 calories per day, which could lead to one pound of weight loss per week, they try dropping 2,000 or more, which is a direct route to metabolic shutdown. For some people, dropping 1,000 calories a day may work, but all weight loss is not created equal. I'll work with you to find that perfect number. Again, I highly recommend you exercise for health, stress relief, and enjoyment. Just don't do it to shed pounds. And if you're overweight or obese, it's probably best for you stay out of the gym to begin with and just do what you're meant to do—eat healthily and walk. You must divorce the idea of exercising to lose weight. You will exercise for health and use proper nutrition to shed the pounds.

If you're serious about losing weight, there are other more important things you must do. Instead of running to the gym for spinning or boot camp, run to your grocery store and arm yourself with healthy food. Start cooking more at home and plan your meals. Eat breakfast and don't skip meals. Practice eating with elegance and don't swear off the foods you love. Get plenty of sleep and manage your stress. These are all ideas we've reviewed in prior chapters, and as I'll explain, they are more important practices than exercise when it comes to shedding pounds.

When you exercise, you think about it only for the half hour or hour that you do it. But food is being consumed all day. And when we diet, we think about it all day long, like what snack to eat, what healthy lunch options are available to us. If we became moderately more active by adding more activity to our everyday life, it has more of an effect than expending a half hour at the gym. I'm talking about things like taking the stairs, biking to work, or parking farther away in the parking lot. You don't have to run a marathon to see positive results in your weight-loss efforts.

So now, let's put these ideas in the context of real clients I've helped by evaluating and reshaping their understanding of how to exercise most effectively for weight loss.

Julia: The Bootcamp Blues

Julia, a 5'8" forty-year-old woman, came to me weighing 200 pounds. On our first appointment, she told me she'd been going to the gym with girlfriends and had signed up for an intensive boot camp. By her own admission, she was not an athlete nor did she follow a regular fitness routine prior to signing up for the program. Once she explained her plan, I commended her for embracing fitness and encouraged her efforts. Julia's mind was made up: she was going to lose weight through the boot camp. Because she had signed up for the program, she had come to the conclusion that she was now very quickly on her way to weight loss.

Once she began exercising, she often complained about how hungry she was and said that her eating plan was not giving her enough calories. She also noted she had intense sugar cravings. So she decided to eat more based on her trainer's recommendations. As time passed, she built up an impressive fitness level, but unfortunately, she hadn't lost any weight. As a matter of fact, she gained two pounds. Her trainer told her that it was muscle and that muscle weighs more than fat. Finally, she revealed that at times she felt she worked out so hard that she was deserving of chocolate chip cookies as a reward. This is a typical story I've seen with so many of my clients. So what was wrong with Julia's approach?

First, Julia is female, so exercising caused her ghrelin levels to spike; she was experiencing true hunger. Because of the intense hunger, she could not sustain the optimal deficit prescribed for her weight loss. In short, her metabolic balance was completely off. Second, a ghrelin spike will make you want to eat as though you are emotionally hungry, which means that food is perceived as very rewarding. This is why Julia craved the chocolate chip cookies. Third, Julia took her exercise to a point that made it difficult to stick to her optimal deficit. Of course, it seems that if you exercise more than you should, you'd be able to eat more, but in my years of experience, it doesn't work out this way. It's more effective to stick to your optimal deficit and maintain the right amount of exercise so that you can control hunger and lose the weight. Since Julia wanted to lose weight instead of gaining muscle, I advised her to slow down on her exercise and to focus on the Eating Free principles.

Julia's story is typical. We all think that upon exercising, even in mild ways or insignificant increments, we have earned the right to eat more food, and often we allow ourselves fatty and sugary foods as a reward for our work. Julia was doing this and yet still feeling hungry because of her poor food choices. Weight loss is as much about the psychological behaviors that accompany our eating, and one of the biggest reasons that exercise should *not* be our primary weight-loss tool is because it often alters our eating behaviors. In the end, and to her credit, Julia resolved to finish the camp. However, she still believed she would lose the weight that way, and sadly, she only gained weight. When she completed boot camp, she had gained an additional two pounds. Finally, she accepted that she needed to give in to the process, so she began the Eating Free program and eventually lost forty pounds.

Now, let's take an example from the other end of the spectrum: a dedicated athlete named Bruce who fell victim to all the most common weight-loss myths.

Bruce: A Spare Tire Despite Eating "Right"

Bruce was a 5'10" forty-six-year-old man who came to me with the goal of losing excess weight. A consummate gym rat, Bruce worked out at least five times a week, if not every day. He hired trainers, used weights, and logged at least four to five hours of cardio work a week. Additionally, he scrutinized every morsel of food he ingested in hopes of sculpting the ideal body. Unfortunately, he bought into every food myth out there, and ate all the wrong things in all the wrong ways. He also believed he could lose fat and gain muscle at the same time, which is a common misconception. Losing weight is a catabolic state while gaining muscle is an anabolic state. If you're building muscle while exercising, it's because you're eating too much. If you are on a caloric deficit, you should be losing fat, not building muscle. That's not something we need to delve into too deeply here, but it's important to understand that you can't do both at once. Anyway, regardless of all the time and energy Bruce devoted to his fitness and nutrition regimen, he carried extra fat around his midsection that he found virtually impossible to lose. By the time he came to see me, he had chalked "the spare tire" up to middle age and just accepted it as his permanent condition. In reality, Bruce was eating "right" in terms of overexercising and undereating. He was also creating more hunger by eating unbalanced combinations of food types or "fake" foods like protein bars.

Bruce discovered my services through a brochure at his gym, and while reading it, he learned about my 80/20 Rule (80 percent nutrition and 20 percent exercise). While he monitored his food intake closely, it had never occurred to him to seek out a registered dietitian because he worked out so intensely. He'd invested hundreds, even thousands of dollars in his fitness efforts, but he could not buy a way to lose that belly fat through his intensive workouts. So we reduced his number of workout days from six to three per week and refocused his attention on approaching weight loss through a smart, informed, nutritional approach.

On his first visit to my office, Bruce weighed in at 193 pounds, with a waist circumference of thirty-seven inches. He had a body fat content of 20 percent, which for most of us would be a desirable enough percentage, but I knew that as a male dedicated to weight training, Bruce's body fat should have been somewhere between 10 to 12 percent. Because he was a highly motivated and disciplined individual, it wasn't hard to help him reach his goal (within six months, he went down to 168 pounds with 11 percent body fat). What *was* difficult was rewiring Bruce's brain about how to get there. He had been following a number of misguided assumptions about protein loading and carb avoidance that were like scripture to him. Science dictates that you need carbs to burn fat, period. If you have too much protein along with too much fat, you'll exceed the number of calories you're able to work off. Getting Bruce to trust me on these matters was the ultimate challenge, as it was a real struggle for him to let go of everything he'd always been told at the gym.

It's important to note that his amazing transformation didn't involve drastically changing his workout; it was mainly changing his nutrition. Why did it work? Because Bruce had been laboring under misinformation about how to lose fat. As he likes to say, "I spent thousands of dollars on a trainer, and you whipped me into shape just by eating better." That was four years ago. Today, Bruce is fifty and he's still at 11 percent body fat. Why? Because he learned how to eat properly and maintain his program in a healthy, realistic manner. It's not rocket science; it's just something most people have never been taught. When Bruce came to me, he was operating under a combination of weight-loss myths we've all heard before.

Myth #1: *Work out on an empty stomach to lose fat.* Bruce had grown up with the assumption that snacking was a sign of weakness. Because he believed it was a poor behavior, he broke himself of it years ago, and never allowed himself to snack on food (only fitness bars), even when he was hungry.

Myth #2: *Avoid carbs.* From *The Atkins Diet* to *The Paleo Diet* to the glut of media misinformation on TV, carbs have become public enemy number one. The poor potato, I always say. Humble old rice, the staple food of Asia (the largest continent on the planet), is now a scapegoat for our poor eating habits. Frankly, it's ridiculous.

Myth #3: *Load up on protein.* Like many of his fellow gym buddies, Bruce believed protein should be his lifeblood. And he'd take it in any form he could find it, most of them made in labs: protein shakes, protein powders, protein bars, even a muscle-building liquid supplement common in fitness clubs. This product, by the way, may build muscle, but it's ultra-high in fat content and it's completely unnecessary. An excess of anything (even protein) will turn to fat in the end. And while this supplement may be useful for someone who is trying to bulk up, it has no place in a weight-loss regimen.

When not having manmade protein products, Bruce loaded up on nuts. Again, nuts are great in moderation, but the fat content is off the charts. Most of my clients are shocked to learn that a standard adult serving of almonds—for those trying to lose weight, mind you—is six almonds. That's right; I said 6, not 60, which is closer to the amount we grab in a couple of handfuls. Next time you decide on nuts for a snack, count them. You'll start to see how our eating patterns and portions have spiraled beyond what our bodies really require.

Okay, so now you've heard stories from two ends of the spectrum: a sedentary person who allowed herself permission to binge based on the idea she was exercising effectively, and a hard-core fitness fanatic who still couldn't lose the fat. If you'll indulge me, I'll share a final story that typifies what can happen when exercise is being used as the primary mode of weight loss.

Aaron: Gaining Weight from Extreme Training

Some years ago, I partnered with the San Francisco Foundation for AIDS LifeCycle, a long-distance cycling event that raises money for AIDS research. Today I help the association with teaching their participants about sports nutrition. I take my responsibility as a certified sports dietitian seriously, and I monitor some of the participants' progress closely. In this role, I come into contact with all kinds of ambitious people—some who are semiprofessional athletes, some who have a personal interest in supporting AIDS causes, and many who sign up for the event as a means of losing weight. These are people like Aaron, a three-time triathlete who signed up for events like the Ironman triathlon so he could lose fifty pounds. Unfortunately, he reported that despite his incredible commitment to exercise, he not only kept weight on but actually gained weight! How is it that someone could train, sometimes for months on end, for a 545-mile bike ride and actually *put on* weight? And before you protest, "That's muscle mass!" let me tell you something: Aaron may have added some muscle, but he didn't lose the gut he hoped to "burn" away. Here's what happened.

The LifeCycle event is a seven-day trek with six to seven hours of riding a day. In order to prepare for this grueling endurance test, Aaron started training well in advance. Like most people, he worked during the week so he left his hardcore training for the weekends. He was riding long distances and covering a lot of miles, sometimes burning as many as 3,000 calories on training events! Sounds incredible, right? You'd think he must have been wasting away to nothing! Wrong. Because of the incredible outpouring of effort, not to mention the psychological effect of exerting so much energy, Aaron gave himself the green light to eat after completing his training events. After his long rides, he tended to eat whatever he wanted—he had earned it, right? And he was famished. And really, who could blame him? We're taught to reward hard work. *Work hard; play hard*, or so the saying goes.

What happened with Aaron was that he should have been fueling while training, but instead he pushed himself without taking the time to eat what his body needed when it was critical. By depriving himself of the essential food his workouts demanded, his body shut down and his metabolism slowed in order to hang on to everything that was stored up in reserve. Then, when the practice events were over, he went nuts around food. After following this weekly pattern, which was also confused with a number of myth-based eating edicts (no carbs, all protein, fitness bars), and then exerting himself like crazy during training, his body went berserk. After these events, he would consume madly. And that was, of course, his downfall.

Many times after training, event coordinators encouraged celebratory outings that were meant to reward riders for their hard work. These came in the form of visiting places that sold cheeseburgers, pizza, burritos, beers, and desserts—sometimes all at once. For Aaron and many of his fellow participants, the training was only on weekends, but the bingeing may have carried on for a few days into the week. And again, let's think about the foods they were eating. Sure, Aaron may have burned 3,000 calories in a weekend, but a couple of waffle and pancake breakfasts or a few doughnuts later, and he'd consumed double, even triple that number of calories.

Also, the practice events were set up on courses lined with stands that invited riders to stop and snack. These stands often include cookies, pasta, sugary energy drinks, and other weight-loss foes. The takeaway from all of this is that long-distance events are a wonderful experience— for bonding, fitness, and charitable causes. But they are not a reliable or recommended way for losing weight. I can't tell you how many clients come to me saying they've signed up to do a marathon or a triathlon as their means of kick-starting their weight loss. If you enjoy these activities, do them for that reason, but be careful about telling yourself you will lose weight—in practice this rarely, if ever, works.

If I've said it once, I've said it a thousand times: Working out should happen on a moderate, regular schedule that's easy enough to maintain with your everyday lifestyle and activities. For most people, that's maybe an hour three times a week. Add up those calories burned and compare them to a week's worth of calories consumed. Chances are they're not going to balance out.

Now that I've illustrated a number of examples about ineffective exercising for weight loss, how do you actually achieve your goal? This is where the 80/20 Rule (80 percent nutrition, 20 percent exercise) comes in. This is not a rule that is quantifiable by caloric equation. It's not a ratio of food intake to energy output. It's a ratio of your effort toward weight loss. What that means is in today's media-obsessed society, we're led to believe we should put 80 percent of our energy toward weight loss into exercise. To make a major shift, you need to dedicate 80 percent of your energy to nutrition if you really hope to lose weight. I still advocate that 20 percent of your efforts go to exercise, but that's a big change from what you're used to hearing. It's a whole new set of priorities, and they involve a time commitment.

Lots of people make time to fit exercise into their busy schedules. They'll put it on their calendars, make appointments with fitness trainers, give up lunch at work, take the kids to day care—all just to exercise. They'll sacrifice for that part of their lives. But when it comes to nutrition, they'll ignore it almost entirely by eating on the go, buying prepackaged foods, picking up lunch or dinner at drive-through fast-food joints, grabbing snacks at the corner coffee shop, or eating standing up or while walking to a meeting.

Exercise Adds Very Little to Your Weight-Loss Equation

Your body works on a weekly average, so exercise adds very little to the equation. Say you take a spinning class two times a week, use weights three times a week, and jog once a week (as shown in Chart 1 below). You can see how many calories are burned in total for the week—in this case 1,900 calories—which sounds like a lot! However, if you divide that number by seven, representing the seven days of the week, you've only burned (or "earned") an extra 271 calories per day.

CHART 1

EXERCISE	CALORIES BURNED/HOUR	FREQUENCY/WEEK	CALORIES
Spinning	400	2	800
Weights	200	3	600
Jog	500	1	500
		Total:	1900
		Average/day	271

CHART 2

RUN	500	500/7	71 CAL

In the second chart, say you add an extra run to your regimen, think-ing it will allow you to have an extra meal out or something. That run will burn 500 calories. Again—divide that over seven days—and you'll really only burn 71 calories a day, which would allow you to eat, say, one extra apple. So if you want to run because it feels good, go for it. But if you think you need to go for a run so you can eat a pizza and drink a six-pack tonight, forget about it.

Recommendations

Exercise is for enjoyment. Don't exercise as punishment for hav-ing body fat. And the worst possible offender: Do *not* exercise to give yourself permission to eat. If you play that card, you've already lost the weight-loss game.

Don't exercise too much or too little. Find the sweet spot so you can follow the caloric prescription given to you. It should feel enjoyable and rewarding. It should leave you refreshed, not wiped out. Many researchers believe that very frequent, low-level physical activity—the kind humans performed for thousands of years before we invented gyms—was actually better for us than the intensive grind we put our-selves through today. What you'll want to do is total the calories you're burning for one week (with actual exercise, not lifestyle activities) and divide it by 7. With that number in mind, remember that I recommend burning no more than 400 calories a day for women and no more than 500 calories a day for men. These amounts will keep your metabolism in check and won't disrupt your ability to stick to your optimal deficit. Stick with this plan and you'll find your hunger is controllable and you'll lose the weight. I do not recommend attempting to lose weight while training for competitions like marathons, cycling events, or the Iron-man. If you're participating in these types of events, fueling right and increasing your performance should be your priority. My recommendations are based on study from my practice and proven success stories.

Be realistic about your time. If you can only exercise three times a week, that's great. Better to be more active throughout the day than to spend an hour on the treadmill. Simple things like walking to the corner store, taking the stairs, and parking at the far end of the lot can make a difference in terms of establishing more regular healthy patterns. Keep it mild—I recommend 150 minutes of moderate cardiovascular per *week*, not per day, as well as supplemental strength training three times a week for 30 minutes to minimize muscle breakdown as much as possible.

Remember the importance of eating before and after exercise. Think in terms of eating more, not less. A good pre-exercise meal for one hour at the gym is a banana with low-fat cheese or Greek yogurt. In the morning, your post-exercise meal would be your actual breakfast, or at night it could be your dinner.

Chapter 11

Your Secret Weapon: The FreeQ (*F*ood, *R*EST, *E*nergy *E*xpenditure Quotient)

AS YOU KNOW, LOSING WEIGHT IS NOT ONLY about reducing calorie intake. Recent research shows us that there is a holistic component of self-care that involves every aspect of our well-being: physical, emotional, psychological—it all adds up to healthy eating for weight loss. One of the things that makes my Eating Free plan unique is that I've developed a tool that helps you track—at any given time—how well you're eating free. Because so many factors influence ghrelin production, it's important to have a constant sense of how well you're balancing the myriad factors that contribute to weight gain—and loss. The tool I am introducing is called the FreeQ, which you can think of as your weight-loss IQ. It's a dynamic tool that scores your current ability to lose weight based on a delicate balance of life factors. Remember, weight loss is a complex equation that works best when everything is in balance. That's where FreeQ comes in. In simple terms, FreeQ stands for:

Food

REST

Energy **E**xpenditure

Quotient

Your FreeQ will give you a complete picture of where you are on any given week. When you score within the desired zone, that means you're eating free and all of your lifestyle factors are currently optimal for weight loss. When your FreeQ score dips into the less-desirable zones, you may be cutting calories, but other factors can conspire to inhibit your weight loss.

The FreeQ is a tool I developed to measure how close you are to entering the Eating Free Zone. This zone is crucial to losing weight effectively. Sure, you can lose weight by just counting calories, but it's not the most effective, sustainable way to achieve your goals.

> By learning how to improve your FreeQ score, you change behaviors that lead you to sustainable success. What you learn is not a plan or a diet. It's a way to live for the rest of your life.

The FreeQ incorporates many aspects into your life that affect your food choices, how you lose weight, how and when you get hungry, the quality of your food, and when and what you eat, as well as how you prepare it. By learning how to improve your FreeQ score, you change behaviors that lead you to sustainable success. What you learn is not a plan or a diet. It's a way to live for the rest of your life. It's the same way that you learn life lessons. For example, I remember my mother telling me never to touch a hot iron. She could tell me a thousand times, but it never sunk in until I touched it. Once I knew what it felt like, that lesson was ingrained in me forever. This is an extreme example, and a negative one, which is not my intent. The point is, people can tell you lots of things about losing weight that go in one ear and out the other, but once you apply the FreeQ and monitor it over a period of time, the principles it teaches will become ingrained and second nature to you.

One thing my clients like about the FreeQ is that it's dynamic. It's a snapshot of your weight-loss potential in any given week. The good news is, if you get a low FreeQ score, it doesn't live on forever. You can drastically improve your score the next week just by applying the principles you'll be learning, many of which are as simple as eating breakfast earlier, adding more snacks, or mixing up your vegetable selection. Your ability to improve your FreeQ rests in your hands, and once you start to see changes, you can't help but want to keep improving your score. Now let's take a look at the actual FreeQ tool so you can get a sense of how it works. (*Please note:* you can also go to www.eatingfree.com to use the free FreeQ online tool as well.)

The FreeQ tool will help you see how close you are to eating free. It helps you see the areas in which you're succeeding and those in which you need to improve. Taking the quiz is like weighing yourself. It is best to do it weekly. Progress varies from week to week, so it is important to check in weekly.

1. Start from the top of the quiz and move down.
2. For every statement with which you agree, mark the corresponding box.
3. There are sections of the quiz where you have stand-alone points and others where you need at least four "yes" statements to earn points.

4. The responses are either "yes" or "no." There are no "sometimes," "maybe," or "usually" options.

5. Once you are done evaluating the statements, tally the total points and you'll get your FreeQ score.

6. Take this number and refer to the description of what your FreeQ score means.

				Date	Date	Date	Date
Food		I am eating less and losing weight.	40	❏	❏	❏	❏
		I am varying and eating whole grains most days.	30 *(you need at least 4 to get points)*	❏	❏	❏	❏
		I am eating the rainbow of fruits and vegetables.		❏	❏	❏	❏
		75% of the types of the fats I eat are heart healthy.		❏	❏	❏	❏
		75% of the meats that I eat are very lean.		❏	❏	❏	❏
		I am eating whole/minimally processed foods most of the time.		❏	❏	❏	❏
REST	**Renew**	I take time to relax.	20 *(you need at least 4 to get points)*	❏	❏	❏	❏
		I manage my time well.		❏	❏	❏	❏
		I know my limits to avoid stress.		❏	❏	❏	❏
		I practice deep breathing exercises.		❏	❏	❏	❏
		I practice eating with elegance.		❏	❏	❏	❏
		I eat all food free of guilt.		❏	❏	❏	❏
		I reward myself with things other than food.		❏	❏	❏	❏

			Date	Date	Date	Date
Energize	I hydrate during the day.	25	❏	❏	❏	❏
	I eat breakfast within 1 hour of waking every day.	*(you need at least 4 to get points)*	❏	❏	❏	❏
	I eat every 3-4 hours.		❏	❏	❏	❏
	I combine carbs/protein when eating.		❏	❏	❏	❏
	I eat 70% of my calories before dinnertime.		❏	❏	❏	❏
	I drink less than 7 servings of alcohol per week.		❏	❏	❏	❏
			___	___	___	___
Sleep	I sleep enough to feel good the next day (6-8 hours)	20	❏	❏	❏	❏
			___	___	___	___
	I record my food enough times to see results.	20	❏	❏	❏	❏
			___	___	___	___
Time for You	I plan what I am going to eat in advance.	20 *(you need at least 4 to get points)*	❏	❏	❏	❏
	I grocery shop weekly.		❏	❏	❏	❏
	I prepare most of my meals at home.		❏	❏	❏	❏
	I sit down to eat and take at least 20 min.		❏	❏	❏	❏
	I eat out at restaurants less than five times per week.		❏	❏	❏	❏
			___	___	___	___
Energy Expenditure	I understand my total energy expenditure.	5	❏	❏	❏	❏
			___	___	___	___
	I exercise for health.	20	❏	❏	❏	❏
	Total FreeQ	200	___	___	___	___

> When your FreeQ score is in the ideal range (above at least 180 to 200), that means everything is working optimally for weight-loss success.

As you can see, just like your IQ, the FreeQ is based on a scale from 1 to 200. The Eating Free Zone exists between 180 and 200. That's the best possible scenario. However, people can still lose weight when scoring 140 and above. The FreeQ takes everything into account, including the quality of food you are eating, the care you take in preparing meals, the amount of rest you get, the amount and kind of energy you expend, and the level of stress you experience. This is how we measure all those factors related to your ghrelin production, your appetite, your stress level, and other lifestyle habits. When your FreeQ score is in the ideal range (above at least 180 to 200), that means everything is working optimally for weight-loss success. Here's how the scoring works:

0–115: This is what I call the danger zone. You're gaining weight and you're at risk to develop inflammation, diabetes, heart disease, cancer, or depression. Anyone who falls into this category needs to take action immediately! Eating Free comes to the rescue.

116–179: This is what I consider to be a warning zone, as some behaviors can lead back to the danger zone. In the warning scoring range, you're not losing weight effectively. If you are losing weight, you're at risk to gain weight back because it's not quality weight loss. In this range you need to set goals, and to lose weight you need a FreeQ score of at least 140.

180–200: Congratulations, you're Eating Free! When you fall into this range, you drastically improve your *nutritional quality of life*. You are losing weight and maintaining your loss. You've freed yourself from diets and you are free to enjoy food. You are a champion!

Let's take a look at the FreeQ quiz components. As you can see, figuring out your FreeQ means responding to thirty simple statements. At any given time, you can take this quiz to see where your FreeQ score lands for that week. Your goal should always be to get into the ideal range, but even lower scores can lead to successful weight loss.

While it may seem like common sense that you should sleep a certain number of hours per night and drink a certain amount of water per day—we've heard all this before—it's the *combination* of these kinds of habits that has a powerful effect on weight loss. The FreeQ questions are actually monitoring factors that relate to ghrelin spikes, which can come from eating habits, stress habits, exercise habits, and more. So while no one factor in the FreeQ seems earth-shattering, taken together, these elements represent the secret to real, lasting results. Eating Free allows you to put all of the elements together in a way that creates the perfect balance to successfully lose and keep off the weight. As you've been learning, it's that total balance—the F (Food), the R (Rest), and the EE (Energy Expenditure) that adds up to success.

The truth is, up until now, we've all lived by a "no pain, no gain" adage that tells us if we're not suffering, we're not succeeding. But science is now showing us that slowing down and taking it easy should be taken seriously. We should understand that relaxing in some measure actually and counterintuitively plays a big part in our weight-loss success. We've all heard the topic come up anecdotally when discussing other cultures.

The truth is, up until now, we've all lived by a "no pain, no gain" adage that tells us if we're not suffering, we're not succeeding. But science is now showing us that slowing down and taking it easy should be taken seriously.

How is it that people in so many other countries take a time-out in the middle of the day to cease working and enjoy a long, hot meal and a siesta, but they don't balloon up? How is it that Italians enjoy pasta as a separate course in addition to an entrée and they don't report the same staggering weight gain that we do as a nation? How is it that the United States has a staggering economy and more gyms than any other place on the planet, and yet we are the fattest nation—and growing more obese by the day?

The answer is simple: balance.

It's a cliché here to speak of "the American Dream"—and yet it's a very real part of our collective identity. (I include myself in that "we" now, having lived in the United States for so many years that it has now become my home.) It's a dream founded on the idea of hard work and continual striving for success. And somewhere along the way, we began to glorify hard work to such an extent that we started sacrificing some of our most primal human needs. We decided that slowing down was weak, that eating quickly and *on the go* was a savvy solution, that skipping meals and sleep altogether was a reflection of our willpower, that working late and on weekends and with high stress was the way to get ahead. We learned to multitask. And when we did, we gave up precious hours of sleep, quiet moments of renewal, long, slow meals, and an overall sense of physical, mental, and spiritual balance. After years of this round-the-clock, pushing-ourselves lifestyle, science is now showing us how we're paying for it.

Now you have the knowledge and the tools to make a change. Just remember, slowing down to relax and enjoy yourself should no longer be viewed as laziness or a feel-good mantra; it's an essential component to your overall well-being, which enables you to lose and to maintain a healthy weight.

Once you've reached your weight-loss goals, the Eating Free program makes it easy to recalculate your food prescription so you can maintain what you've achieved.

Maintenance

Finally, the day will arrive when you reach your weight-loss goal—and what a day that will be! All the principles you've learned, all the practices you've adopted, all the strategies you've internalized have now given you a solid foundation for moving forward with a new lifestyle approach to food and eating behaviors. Of course, you won't have to continue to follow your optimal deficit because you will have achieved your goals. What you will need to do is go back to my online tool and recalculate your caloric intake for the day based on a goal of weight maintenance rather than weight loss. That new number will be calculated to support the appropriate energy balance for your new body weight.

Typically, I recommend eating 250 to 300 calories less than your total calories to maintain your new weight. This way, you'll have a buffer window just in case you decide to splurge a bit. So, for example, if your total maintenance calories are 2,200, I'll recommend following a 1,900-calorie plan to be on the safe side.

Remember that through maintenance your weight may fluctuate up and down three pounds day to day, especially if you're a woman. So if you are up more than five pounds, restart your optimum deficit immediately. Continue weighing yourself weekly so you are aware, but don't panic if your weight goes up day to day. Remember, ten pounds means the next-size clothing, so rather than buying the next size, start your weight-loss program again. If you buy the next size, that means ten more pounds.

Finally, I recommend that you continue on with your record keeping for a few weeks at your new maintenance weight. This will help you retrain your eye—and your brain—to instinctively understand your new blend of foods and portion sizes to sustain your goal weight.

Congratulations! You are now eating free! Always remember that eating is for survival—but eating free is your choice.

Chapter 12

Freecipes

Vegetarian Recipes

Asian Noodle Primavera

Serves 4
(1½ cups each)

I love this recipe because it's easy to prepare and it gives you that Asian flair. Sometimes I want noodles, but I'm not in the mood for Italian, which can be heavy. This is a great way to satisfy that craving with more exotic flavors.

14 ounces udon noodles, precooked
¼ cup rice vinegar
¼ cup low-sodium soy sauce
¼ cup water
2 tablespoons brown sugar
½ teaspoon red hot chili pepper flakes
1 tablespoon cornstarch
2 teaspoons olive oil

1 small red onion, cut into ¼-inch
   wedges
1 small yellow bell pepper, sliced
   into strips
8 stalks asparagus, chopped
1 cup sliced shiitake mushrooms
2 small bok choy, chopped
4 green onions, thinly sliced

❶ Heat the udon noodles according to package directions; drain and set aside.

❷ Combine rice vinegar, soy sauce, water, brown sugar, pepper flakes, and cornstarch in a small bowl.

❸ Heat oil in a large pan or wok over medium-high heat. Add red onion, bell pepper, and asparagus and cook; stir constantly for 3 minutes.

❹ Add mushrooms and bok choy; stir for another 3 minutes.

❺ Stir sauce mixture into vegetables and heat until sauce begins to thicken; stir constantly.

❻ Stir in green onions.

❼ Add drained noodles and toss to combine well.

Calories 224; Fat 2.7g; Protein 9.3g; Carb. 45g; Fiber 3.6g; Sugar 11.2g
Freebies: 2 G&S, 2 NSV, 0.5 Fat

Cozy Crockpot Chili

Serves 6
(1 cup each)

This is a recipe that you can assemble in the morning or the night before. When you come home, it will be warm and steamy—ready to eat. Best of all, you'll have leftovers through the week.

2 cups water

1 cup apple juice

1 cup vegetable broth

½ teaspoon dried oregano

½ teaspoon dried thyme

3 tablespoons tomato paste

1 teaspoon ground cumin

⅛ teaspoon cayenne pepper

⅛ teaspoon white pepper

2 medium onions, chopped

3 garlic cloves, minced

2 cans (4-ounce) chopped green
   chilies, drained

2 cans (15-ounce) black beans,
   rinsed and drained

2 red bell peppers, chopped

¼ cup chopped fresh cilantro

❶ Combine all ingredients except cilantro in a 4-quart slow cooker. Cover and cook on low for 8 hours. Stir in the cilantro just before serving.

Calories: 121; Fat 0.3g; Protein 5.8g; Carb. 25g; Fiber 5.8g; Sugar 8.5g
Freebies: 1¼ G&S; 1 NSV

Farro Vegetable Salad

Serves 8
(1 cup each)

Farro has long been a staple in Italy. It's a whole grain similar to barley, and it has become one of my top choices. It's so filling, and I prefer it to pasta in soups and meat dishes. Try it, and I know you'll be sold.

1 tablespoon olive oil	3 tomatoes, chopped
1 small onion, chopped	1 bunch fresh basil, chopped
1 tablespoon crushed garlic clove	4 cups roasted vegetables
4 cups chicken broth	(see recipe, page 208)
2 cups farro, dry uncooked	Salt and pepper (optional)

❶ In a medium-size pot, heat olive oil over medium-low heat. Add onion and garlic; sauté until golden brown.

❷ Add chicken broth and let boil. Then add farro and cook for 20 to 30 minutes. *Note:* Farro cooks like brown rice.

❸ When farro is cooked, add tomatoes, basil, and roasted vegetables; mix.

❹ Add salt and pepper to taste before serving (optional).

Calories: 234; Fat 3.9g; Protein 9.1g; Carb. 44.1g; Fiber 11.1g; Sugar 4.2g
Freebies: 2 G&S; 0.5 Meat; 2 NSV; 0.5 Fat

Roasted Cauliflower Soup

Serves 5
(2 cups each)

This soup is a real winner. The roasting provides a deep flavor, and even people who swear they don't like cauliflower are blown away by how delicious and satisfying this tastes.

2 large cauliflower, florets only

Olive oil spray

2 tablespoons olive oil

1 small yellow onion, chopped

1 tablespoon garlic clove, crushed

5 cups chicken broth

❶ Preheat oven to 400°F.

❷ Clean and break the cauliflower, keeping only the florets.

❸ Spray a roasting pan with olive oil and place the cauliflower florets in the pan. Bake for about 20 minutes or until brown.

❹ In a large pot over medium heat, add the olive oil and sauté the onions and garlic until golden brown.

❺ Add the chicken broth and the roasted cauliflower to the pot and cook for 30 minutes or until the cauliflower is soft.

❻ Lower heat and use a handheld blender or food processor to blend the cauliflower mixture into a soup consistency. If necessary, reheat before serving.

❼ Add salt and pepper to taste.

Calories: 68; Fat 3g; Protein 3.3g; Carb. 9.2g; Fiber 2.7g; Sugar 4.1g
Freebies: 0.5 Meat; 1 NSV; 0.5 Fat

Roasted Vegetables

Serves 12
(1 cup each)

This is similar to a traditional ratatouille, and it is one of my best secret weapons. I use this as a side, in pasta sauces, in salads, on meats—you name it. The combination brings a different dimension to your dishes, and it gives you so many great vegetables. Once you bring this into your recipe list, you'll always go back to it.

Olive oil spray

1 large red onion, cut into
large pieces

2 red bell peppers, cut into large
pieces

4 medium zucchini, cut into large
pieces

1 large eggplant, cut into large
pieces

1 large cauliflower, florets only

A pinch of garlic powder

Salt and black pepper to taste

❶ Preheat oven to 400°F.

❷ Spray a large roasting pan with olive oil.

❸ Place the cut vegetables into the pan, making a single layer, and spray olive oil over them.

❹ Sprinkle garlic powder, salt, and black pepper over the vegetables to taste.

❺ Place roasting pan in the oven for about 20 minutes.

❻ Stir the vegetables and place them back in the oven for another 5 to 10 minutes or until desired color/tenderness (I prefer mine slightly soft and browned).

Calories: 66; Fat 1.6g; Protein 4g; Carb. 11.6g; Fiber 4.6g; Sugar 5.8g
Freebies: 2 NSV; 0.5 FAT

Tuscan White Bean Puree

Serves 6
(½ cup each)

This makes a good dip at parties. Pair it with vegetables or use it on top of meats instead of sauce. It tastes great and it adds some healthy legumes to your meal.

1 tablespoon olive oil

1 cup chopped onions

2 teaspoons crushed garlic clove

2 cans cannellini beans, drained

1 cup vegetable broth

❶ Sauté onion and garlic in olive oil over medium heat until golden brown.

❷ Pour beans into the mixture and sauté.

❸ Add vegetable broth and let simmer for 5 to 10 minutes.

❹ Puree mixture with a handheld blender or in a food processor to the consistency of a dip. Add extra vegetable broth as needed to achieve desired consistency.

❺ Add salt and pepper to taste (optional).

Calories: 150; Fat 2.3g; Protein 9.7g; Carb. 26.4g; Fiber 7.5g; Sugar 3.6g
Freebies: 1 G&S; 1 Meat; 0.5 Fat

Veggie Pizza

Serves 8
(1 slice each)

Who doesn't love pizza? I made this vegetarian to demonstrate that it's easy to get your veggies in a yummy way. However, you can feel free to make it your own by adding meat according to your freebies. Again, this is a great one for the whole family, including kids.

16 ounces whole wheat pizza dough
Cornmeal (for dusting) or
    parchment paper
2 cups low-fat pasta sauce
2 cups raw spinach, roughly
    chopped

1 cup thinly sliced mushrooms
1 cup thinly sliced green bell pepper
½ cup thinly sliced red onion
2 cups of low-fat mozzarella cheese,
    grated

❶ Preheat the oven to 400° F.

❷ Remove the dough from the package. Sprinkle the bottom of a nonstick baking sheet with cornmeal (to prevent the dough from sticking to the baking sheet), then spread the dough across the pan.

❸ Spread the pasta sauce on top.

❹ Spread all of the vegetables over the top of the pasta sauce.

❺ Sprinkle with the shredded low-fat mozzarella.

❻ Bake for 10 to 15 minutes until the cheese is melted.

Calories: 212; Fat 3.6g; Protein 14g; Carb. 34g; Fiber 6.3g; Sugar 5.6g
Freebies: 1.5 G&S; 1.5 Meat; 1 NSV; 0.5 Fat

Zesty Hummus

Serves 5
(4 tablespoons or
¼ cup each)

Often, we think of hummus as a fattening snack food, but this is a tasty, creamy, low-fat version. It's the perfect snack dip for vegetables like baby carrots and celery. And, of course, it's another great way to add powerful nutrition from legumes into your meals. You're going to love it!

2 garlic cloves, minced

¼ teaspoon cumin

¼ teaspoon salt

2 teaspoons lemon juice

1 tablespoon olive oil

1 can garbanzo beans; reserve
   2 tablespoons of the liquid
   and discard the remainder

❶ Combine all ingredients in a blender or food processor and blend until smooth.

Calories: 95; Fat 3g; Protein 4g; Carb. 12g; Fiber 3g; Sugar 1g
Freebies: 1 G&S; 0.5 Meat; 0.5 Fat

Banana Walnut Steel Cut Oatmeal

Serves 6
(½ cup each)

Oatmeal is one of my favorite things to eat for breakfast. I like to make it in advance on the weekends so I can enjoy it all week long. I sweeten it with mashed banana, and it has a great depth of nutty flavor. To me, it tastes like cake—what a treat! Plus, you can add blueberries and flaxseed to make it more flavorful and filling.

4 cups water

3 cinnamon sticks

¼ teaspoon salt

1 cup steel cut oats, dry

4 tablespoons walnuts, chopped

1 banana, medium size, mashed

❶ Boil water with cinnamon and salt. Once water boils, reduce heat. Add oats, walnuts, and banana. Stir and cook over low heat. Stir occasionally. Cook for 25 to 30 minutes.

Note: This recipe can be eaten throughout the week, since it lasts for about five days in the refrigerator.

Calories: 159; Fat 5.2g; Protein 5.5g; Carb. 23.9g; Fiber 6.8g; Sugar 2.5g
Freebies: 1 G&S; 0.5 Meat; 1 Fat

Beef, Pork, Poultry, and Seafood Freecipes

Peruvian Cilantro Beef Stew

Serves 10
(1½ cups each)

This is one of my favorite childhood recipes from Peru. Talk about flavor! It's a great one to make for company, for the whole family, or simply to last all week long. It's another one that leaves great leftovers, and like most stews, it tastes better the next day.

1 tablespoon olive oil

½ medium onion, chopped

2 garlic cloves, minced

1½ pounds raw beef stewing
   meat, very lean

1 teaspoon ground cumin

2 cups canned beef broth

1 bunch cilantro, chopped

3 to 4 small unpeeled red
   potatoes, cubed

½ cup frozen carrots

1 cup frozen green peas

❶ Put two teaspoons of the olive oil into a pan and sauté the onions and garlic over medium-high heat.

❷ Put the remaining olive oil in a separate pan and sear the beef. Reserve the beef juice.

❸ Add the beef and cumin to the onion and garlic mixture. Stir and cook on low heat, then cover.

❹ Meanwhile, put the beef broth and cilantro into a blender and blend. Add to the beef mixture. Cover and simmer on low heat for 30 to 40 minutes.

❺ Add the potatoes and cook for 30 minutes.

❻ Add the carrots and peas and cook for 10 to 15 minutes.

Note: If you're using fresh carrots, add them at the same time you add the potatoes and cook for 30 minutes. Also, in Peruvian culture, you eat this dish with rice and pinto/white beans.

Calories: 183; Fat 5.6g; Protein 22.9g; Carb. 8.9g; Fiber 1.4g; Sugar 1.6g
Freebies: 0.5 G&S; 3 Meat; 1 Fat

Spicy Steak Fajitas

Serves 4
(1 tortilla with
4 ounces of steak/
vegetable mixture
per person)

Most people I know love Mexican food, and this traditional favorite comes alive with spicy flavor. You get all the satisfaction without any unhealthy ingredients.

For marinade:

3 tablespoons lime juice

1 tablespoon olive oil

2 garlic cloves, minced

½ teaspoon ground cumin

1 fresh jalapeño pepper, chopped

½ cup fresh cilantro, chopped

For fajitas:

16 ounces beef skirt steak, lean

1 tablespoon olive oil

1 large yellow onion, sliced into
   ½-inch pieces

1 large green bell pepper, sliced
   into ½-inch pieces

1 large red bell pepper, sliced into
   ½-inch pieces

8 whole wheat tortillas

Salsa, if desired

Nonfat sour cream, if desired

❶ Mix all the ingredients for the marinade together and place with the steak in a large ziplock bag, pressing out as much air as possible. Let steak sit in the refrigerator for at least 1 hour and up to 24 hours (a longer marinating time is better). When ready, remove the steak from the bag and drain.

❷ Slice steak across the grain into finger-length strips. Cook strips in a large pan at high heat, turning frequently, 1½ to 2 minutes (cook in batches, if necessary).

❸ Heat the pan on high and add the remaining tablespoon of olive oil. Quickly stir-fry the onion and bell pepper just until limp, about 3 to 4 minutes.

❹ Heat tortillas in the microwave for 30 seconds. Assemble with steak/vegetable mix and serve with salsa and nonfat sour cream.

Calories: 217; Fat 11.2g; Protein 20.7g; Carb. 14.7g; Fiber 8.1g; Sugar 2.2g
Freebies: 1 G&S; 3 Meat; 2 Fat

Peach Chutney Pork Chops

Serves 4   It may sound fancy, but this dish is easy and scrumptious. What a great alternative to the boring old chicken breast. The great thing is, it's just as lean.

1 pound lean pork loin chops	½ cup peach jelly
Salt, to taste	2 tablespoons Dijon mustard
Pepper, to taste	¼ teaspoon ground ginger
1 tablespoon olive oil	¼ cup cider vinegar or white vinegar

❶ Pat chops dry with a paper towel. Sprinkle salt and pepper on them to marinade.

❷ Heat oil in a large skillet over medium heat. Lightly brown both sides of the pork chops for about 1 to 2 minutes each side.

❸ While the pork chops are cooking, mix the jelly, mustard, and ginger together in a small bowl. Once the chops are almost done, reduce the heat to low. Dollop the sauce over the chops.

❹ Cover the skillet and cook for about 5 to 10 minutes or until the chops are cooked thoroughly.

❺ Remove the chops from the skillet and place on a plate, leaving the remaining sauce in the skillet. Add vinegar and increase the heat to high. Boil down the sauce, scraping up the brown bits from the bottom of the pan.

❻ Add any juices that have come out of the chops while sitting on the plate to the sauce. Mix in thoroughly.

❼ Serve the chops with the sauce.

Calories: 274; Fat 6g; Protein 25.4g; Carb. 26.2g; Fiber 0g; Sugar 24.1g
Freebies: 3.5 Meat, 1 Fat; 1.5 Sugar

Pork Adobo

Serves 4 Like Latin flair? This dish brings great flavor with the adobo prep-aration. If you're not familiar with adobo, I assure you, you'll want to add it to your repertoire when you want an extra flavorful kick.

3 tablespoons paprika

1 teaspoon black pepper

1 teaspoon salt

1½ teaspoons chili powder

1 tablespoon brown sugar

½ teaspoon red chili pepper flakes

1 pound lean pork tenderloin chop

❶ Preheat oven to 400°F.

❷ In a small bowl, combine paprika, pepper, salt, chili powder, brown sugar, and red chili pepper flakes. Rub pork pieces with seasoning mix and coat well.

❸ Preheat skillet to medium-high heat and pan sear the pork on both sides to brown the outside. Transfer the pork to an oven-safe dish and bake for 20 minutes or until an internal temperature reaches 165 degrees.

❹ Remove the pork from the oven and let stand for 5 minutes. Serve with your choice of side dish.

Calories: 188; Fat 6.9g; Protein 25.8g; Carb. 6g; Fiber 2.4g; Sugar 2.9g
Freebies: 3.5 Meat; 1.5 Fat

Asian Chicken Vegetable Stir-Fry

Serves 4
(1 cup each)

It really doesn't get any easier than a traditional stir-fry. It's all the comfort of a sizzling hot meal in only minutes.

1 tablespoon olive oil

2 garlic cloves, minced

1 pound skinless and boneless
   chicken breast, diced

1 teaspoon ground pepper
   (optional)

1 cup snap peas

1 cup sliced mushrooms

1 cup bean sprouts

1 tablespoon low-sodium soy sauce

1 tablespoon rice vinegar

1 tablespoon hot sauce (optional)

❶ Heat 2 teaspoons of oil in a pan or wok over medium-high heat. Add half the garlic and lightly brown.

❷ Add the chicken and the black pepper. Cook for about 5 minutes or until done. Remove from the pan and set chicken aside.

❸ Heat the remaining teaspoon of oil in a pan or wok over medium-high heat. Add remaining garlic and lightly brown.

❹ Add snap peas and cook for 2 minutes. Add mushrooms and bean sprouts and cook for 1 minute.

❺ Reduce heat to medium low. Add the chicken, soy sauce, rice vinegar, and hot sauce (if desired) and stir-fry for about 2 to 3 minutes.

❻ Turn off heat and serve over ½ or 1 cup brown rice.

Calories: 214; Fat 4.9g; Protein 29.5g; Carb. 11g; Fiber 1.9g; Sugar 6.6g
Freebies: 4 Meat; 0.5 NSV; 1 Fat

BBQ Chicken Sandwich

Serves 4

When you're too tired to cook, why not just assemble sand-wiches? This is a great one to make with children, and the prepared chicken makes it a snap.

5 cups skinless rotisserie chicken, white meat only, shredded

½ cup barbecue sauce

½ cup pickled jalapeño pepper slices, drained

4 whole wheat hamburger buns

2 tomatoes, sliced

4 leaves Romaine lettuce

❶ Combine chicken, BBQ sauce, and jalapeños in a large bowl.

❷ Divide the mixture evenly among the bottoms of the buns.

❸ Divide the tomato slices and lettuce leaves among the buns, then put the tops of the buns over the bottoms.

❹ Serve with a side of dill pickles (optional).

Calories: 330; Fat 7g; Protein 30.2g; Carb. 36g; Fiber 4g; Sugar 5.6g
Freebies: 2 G&S; 3.5 Meat; 1 NSV; 1 Fat; 0.5 Sugars

Heart-Healthy Turkey Meatloaf

Serves 8   I love to serve this comfort food favorite with any number of vegetables, plus mashed potatoes, quinoa, or brown rice. I also pair it with my Tuscan White Bean Puree (recipe is included on p. 209).

½ cup chopped onions	¼ cup raw egg whites
½ cup chopped celery	¼ cup 1% milk
½ cup chopped carrots	⅛ cup ketchup
1½ pounds extra lean ground turkey	1 raw egg
⅓ cup flaxseed meal	½ can tomato sauce (7.5 ounce)

❶ Preheat oven to 350°F.

❷ Place chopped onion, celery, and carrots into a food processor and grind.

❸ Combine vegetable mixture with all other ingredients in a bowl and add salt and pepper to taste.

❹ Pour final mixture into a meatloaf dish or shape into a log on a baking sheet and place in oven for 45 minutes.

❺ Slice and serve.

Calories: 145; Fat 3g; Protein 23.9g; Carb. 6.6g; Fiber 2.4g; Sugar 3.9g
Freebies: 3.5 Meat; 1 NSV; 0.5 Fat

Indian Chicken Mango Curry

Serves 4
(1 cup each)

Just because you're eating healthy doesn't mean your food needs to be bland. This dish brings all the exotic spices of India to your table in a fairly easy recipe. It's the perfect introduction to cooking foods from faraway lands.

Sauce:
3 tablespoons tomato paste
2 tablespoons nonfat plain yogurt
1 tablespoon garam masala powder
1 pinch cayenne pepper
1 garlic clove, crushed
2 tablespoons mango chutney
½ teaspoon salt

Chicken:
1 tablespoon olive oil
1 pound skinless, boneless
    chicken, cubed
⅔ cup water
2 serrano chilies, chopped (optional)
2 tablespoons chopped fresh
    cilantro (optional)

❶ Combine sauce ingredients in a bowl.

❷ Heat olive oil on medium in a deep frying pan. Pour the sauce into the pan and bring to a boil. Lower heat and cook for 2 minutes, stirring frequently.

❸ Add the chicken pieces and stir until they are well coated.

❹ Add the water to the pan. Continue to simmer on medium for 5 to 7 minutes, until the chicken is tender.

❺ Add the fresh chilies and cilantro and cook for 2 minutes.

❻ Serve over brown basmati rice.

Calories: 208; Fat 7.5g; Protein 26g; Carb. 8.2g; Fiber 0.8g; Sugar 4.9g
Freebies: 3.5 Meat; 1.5 Fat; 0.5 Sugar

Classic Linguine with Clams

Serves 6
(1 cup each)

This is for the seafood lover who likes a little pasta too. A very clean and elegant recipe, it makes a perfect dish to serve to company while still sticking to a healthy Eating Free program.

1 box linguine pasta, uncooked

1 tablespoon olive oil

4 garlic cloves, minced

2 cans (10 ounces each) baby clams, drained with juice reserved

½ cup white wine

½ cup diced tomatoes (canned, no salt added)

½ teaspoon black pepper

½ teaspoon crushed red chili pepper flakes

½ bunch fresh basil, chopped roughly

❶ Cook pasta according to the directions on the box, then drain.

❷ Meanwhile, heat the olive oil in the pan on low heat. Add the garlic and cook 1 to 2 minutes.

❸ Add the reserved clam juice and white wine. Stir in tomatoes, black pepper, and red chili pepper flakes.

❹ Bring to a boil, reduce heat, and simmer for about 3 minutes. Add clams and cook for 1 minute to warm thoroughly.

❺ Serve over pasta and sprinkle with basil.

Calories: 265; Fat 4.3g; Protein 10.4g; Carb. 44.2g; Fiber 3.8g; Sugar 5.2g
Freebies: 2 G&S; 0.5 Meat, 1 Fat

Oven-Baked Fish Fillets

Serves 4

We love cooking fish in a healthy way, so if you're craving fish and chips, this is the ticket. Forget frozen fish sticks; this gives the same satisfaction in a homemade version you're going to love.

½ teaspoon salt

¼ teaspoon black pepper

¼ teaspoon paprika

½ cup low-fat plain yogurt

1 cup Japanese-style bread crumbs
(panko or similar)

1 pound fish fillets

3 sprays olive oil cooking spray

❶ Preheat oven to 400°F. Place oven rack at the top of the oven.

❷ Add salt, pepper, and paprika to yogurt. Place the bread crumbs in a bowl. Dip the fish in the yogurt mixture, then into the bread crumbs to coat.

❸ Arrange the fish 2 inches apart in a shallow baking pan and spray evenly with 3 sprays (1 second total) of olive oil, just to coat lightly.

❹ Place fish in the oven and bake until surface is well browned.

Note: If fish has not completely cooked by the time the surface has browned, reduce heat to 350°F and continue to bake, checking after 5 minutes or until flesh is flaky.

Calories: 231; Fat 8g; Protein 25.2g; Carb. 12.5g; Fiber 0.7g; Sugar 2.7g
Freebies: 1 G&S; 3.5 Meat; 1.5 Fat

Salmon Salad

Serves 6

In this recipe, I substitute omega-3-rich salmon in place of traditional tuna. It elevates the dish, and it couldn't be better for you. Plus, of course, it tastes divine.

10 ounces canned salmon,
    bones removed
1 tablespoon lime juice
1 tablespoon capers

¼ cup chopped red onions
2 teaspoons olive oil
Salt and pepper to taste

❶ Mix all ingredients together and add salt and pepper to taste. *Note:* Add salmon to a salad, make a sandwich or wrap with it, or pair it with whole wheat crackers.

Calories: 91; Fat 4.2g; Protein 12.8g; Carb. 0.8g; Fiber 0g; Sugar 0g
Freebies: 2 Meat; 1 Fat

Thai Soy Cilantro Fish

Serves 4

This is so simple, with so few ingredients. It's all about the freshness and a taste that will transport you to Southeast Asia.

1 pound fish fillets

1 bunch cilantro, chopped

4 garlic cloves, minced

1 tablespoon maple syrup

6 tablespoons low-sodium
   soy sauce

❶ Place all ingredients in a large ziplock bag. Toss and mix together to evenly coat fish.

❷ Marinate in the refrigerator for at least 20 minutes.

❸ Preheat oven to 400°F.

❹ Spray a shallow baking pan or cookie sheet with olive oil and place the fish fillets on it. Pour any leftover marinade over the fish.

❺ Bake for about 10 to 12 minutes, or until fish is flaky. When done, remove from oven and serve.

Calories: 108; Fat 2.5g; Protein 15.8g; Carb. 5.9g; Fiber 0.5g; Sugar 2.5g
Freebies: 2.5 Meat; 0.5 Fat; 0.5 Sugar

Louisiana Jambalaya

Serves 8
(1 cup each)

I love New Orleans and nothing captures the amazing spirit and Cajun culture of that amazing city like one of its most traditional dishes. This one will definitely put you in a party mood.

1½ cups uncooked rice

1 pound medium-size shrimp,
  no shell and deveined

2 links Cajun Andouille chicken
  sausage, chopped

1 cup finely chopped bell peppers

½ cup finely chopped onion

2 celery stalks, chopped finely

1 cup sliced mushrooms

2 cups beef broth

1 tablespoon olive oil

1 teaspoon paprika

1 teaspoon cayenne pepper

1 teaspoon onion powder

1 teaspoon garlic powder

❶ Rinse the rice with water 2 to 3 times; drain water. Add 1½ cups of water and the remaining ingredients to the rice and cook in a rice cooker or put ingredients into a pot on the stovetop. Bring to a boil. Reduce heat to a simmer. Cover and cook for about 20 to 25 minutes. When the rice is finished, toss and fluff before eating.

Calories: 281; Fat 5.1g; Protein 24.1g; Carb. 33.4g; Fiber 2.2g; Sugar 1.6g
Freebies: 2 G&S; 3 Meat; 0.5 NSV; 1 Fat

Sweet Sautéed Shrimp

Serves 4 Don't be fooled by the word "ketchup" in the recipe—this is not your standard high-fructose corn syrup ketchup. It's an organic version store-bought that's better for you, and kids love it, too.

1 pound large raw shrimp

1 tablespoon olive oil

1 tablespoon garlic clove, chopped

1 tablespoon ginger, chopped

3 tablespoons organic ketchup

1 tablespoon low-sodium soy sauce

2 teaspoons maple syrup

Hot sauce (optional)

❶ Clean and remove the shells from the shrimp.

❷ Heat oil in pan over medium-high heat. Sauté garlic and ginger until golden brown.

❸ Add the shrimp and cook for about 1 to 2 minutes. Reduce heat to medium low.

❹ Add the ketchup, soy sauce, and maple syrup. *Optional:* Add hot sauce if desired. Mix, sauté, and cook for about 1 to 2 minutes.

❺ Turn heat off and serve.

Calories: 176; Fat 5.4g; Protein 23.6g; Carb. 7.5g; Fiber 0g; Sugar 4.7g
Freebies: 3.5 Meat; 1 Fat; 0.5 Sugar

Easy Beef Lasagna

Serves 8
(1 square, about 312 grams)

Lasagna is a home-cooked dish that grandmothers always make, but it always seems to take a long time to prepare. This recipe delivers the taste of Grandma's lasagna with less hassle and less time. I used fewer pasta sheets per layer to make it less carb dense and leaner meat to make it lower in fat.

1 tablespoon olive oil	24 ounces marinara sauce, jarred or canned
1 medium onion, chopped	(choose a marinara sauce that contains
4 garlic cloves, chopped	less than 2 grams of fat and 3 grams of
1 pound ground beef	sugar per serving)
(97% lean and 3% fat)	2 cups (about 16 ounces) tomato sauce,
1 teaspoon salt	canned
1 teaspoon black pepper	4 cups mozzarella cheese, reduced 2% milk
1 tablespoon dried oregano	10 sheets lasagna pasta, no boiling required

❶ Heat 1 tablespoon of oil in pan over medium-high heat. Sauté garlic and onion in oil for about 2-3 minutes.

❷ Once the garlic and onion are lightly browned, add ground beef, salt, pepper and oregano. Cook until browned and crumbled. Mix well.

❸ Add marinara sauce and 1 cup of tomato sauce to beef mixture. Stir and let simmer for about 10 minutes on medium-low heat.

❹ While the mixture is simmering, preheat the oven to 375°F. Then spray a baking pan, about 13x9x3 inches deep, with nonstick cooking oil.

❺ Once the meat sauce mixture is done simmering, turn the heat off.

❻ Mix ½ cup of tomato sauce with 2 ounces of water. Then pour onto the bottom of the baking pan.

❼ Layer 3 uncooked sheets; place 2 lasagna sheets horizontally on the left side of the pan and 1 sheet vertically on the right side. Add half the meat sauce and 1½ cups of cheese on top.

❽ Layer 3 uncooked sheets; place 1 lasagna sheet vertically on the left side of the pan and 2 sheets horizontally on the right side. Add the other half of the meat sauce and 1½ cups of cheese on top.

❾ Layer 4 uncooked sheets: place 4 lasagna sheets vertically. Mix ½ cup of tomato sauce and 2 ounces of water and spread evenly on top of lasagna sheets. Finally, add 1 cup of cheese evenly on top.

❿ Cover baking pan with aluminum foil. Bake for 50 minutes. Remove foil and continue to bake for about 10 minutes to brown the cheese.

⓫ Turn oven off, remove lasagna from oven, let stand for 10 minutes and enjoy.

Calories: 367; Fat 14g; Protein 26.5g; Carbs 32g; Fiber 4g; Sugar 6.2g
Freebies: 1.5 G&S; 3 Meat; 2.7 Fat; 1 NSV

Dessert Recipes

Abuela's Rice Pudding

Serves 10
(½ cup each)

As the name suggests, this was my grandmother's rice pudding recipe. I can't even tell you how much this takes me back to my childhood. The smells, the texture, the taste—it's simply divine. I promise you will love it as much as I do.

1 cup rice, uncooked
3 cups water
Orange peel from ½ orange
2 cinnamon sticks
5 cloves

Salt, to taste
1 12-ounce can 2% evaporated milk
1 12-ounce can sweetened condensed milk

❶ In a large pot over medium-low heat, add rice, water, orange peel, cinnamon sticks, cloves, and salt. Bring to a boil, then reduce heat, cover, and simmer for 15 to 20 minutes. The rice must be well cooked (nicely chewy and tender); test by trying a grain.

❷ Remove from heat and take out the orange peel, cinnamon sticks, and cloves.

❸ Add the evaporated and sweetened condensed milk. Bring to a boil over low heat for about 10 minutes. Stir constantly with a wooden spoon, and the mixture will thicken. Once it has thickened to the desired consistency, remove from heat and serve.

Calories: 133; Fat 1.5g; Protein 4.2g; Carb. 21.8g; Fiber 0.8g; Sugar 5.8g
Freebies: 0.5 G&S; 0.5 Milk; 0.5 Sugar

Applesauce Agave Banana Bread

Serves 16
(1 slice, about 74 grams)

Banana bread is a traditional favorite. By substituting agave nectar for sugar and applesauce for oil, you can enjoy this sweet treat with less sugar, less fat—and no guilt. Your children will love it!

3 medium bananas, ripe

½ cup agave nectar

½ cup applesauce

1 teaspoon vanilla extract

2 eggs, raw

1 teaspoon baking soda

1 teaspoon baking powder

1 teaspoon salt

2 cups flour

❶ Preheat the oven to 325°F. Place the bananas in a large bowl and mash with an electric mixer. Stir in the agave nectar and let stand for 15 minutes. Note: Because agave nectar has a lower glycemic index than sugar, less agave nectar is used and it browns sooner, which is why the bread is baked at a lower temperature for a longer time.

❷ Add the applesauce and eggs and beat well. Add the remaining ingredients and mix thoroughly. Pour into a 9"x5" loaf pan coated with nonstick vegetable spray. Bake for about 75 minutes, or until a wooden toothpick inserted in the center of the loaf comes out clean. Note: every oven is different, so total baking time may vary. Use a toothpick at 60 minutes to check doneness of bread.

❸ Remove from the oven and let stand for 10 minutes before removing from the pan. Cool on a wire rack.

Calories: 120; Fat1g; Protein 2.7g; Carb. 26g; Fiber 1g; Sugar 11.8g
Freebies: 1 G&S; 0.4 Fruit; 0.4 Sugar

Decadent Chocolate Figs

Serves 12
(1 chocolate-covered fig, about 27 grams)

Sweet tooth, anyone? This recipe brings together three of nature's best offerings: sweet fruit, dark chocolate, and powerful antioxidants.

1 bar (about 100 grams) dark chocolate, 73% dark

(Chocolate per 100g Fat 36g; Carb. 45g; Fiber 12g; Sugars 27g; Protein 6g)

12 (about 227g) dried figs, Mission or Calimyrna

❶ Chop chocolate in even pieces to make it easier to melt. Place in a stainless steel bowl.

❷ Add two to three inches of water to a pot. Bring water into a simmer and turn off heat.

❸ Place bowl of chocolates on top of the simmering water. Note: avoid water going into the chocolate; they do not mix well. Also, make sure the bowl does not touch the water, leaving 1-2 inches between the water and bowl. The steam from the simmering water is sufficient to melt the chocolate.

❹ Stir the chocolate constantly to ensure even melting. By keeping the heat very low and constantly stirring, you can always melt without overheating.

❺ When you see the chocolate is almost melted, remove the bowl from the simmering pot of water and stir until smooth and shiny.

❻ Then dip figs into the melted dark chocolate, covering the fig completely. Place figs on a sheet of parchment or wax paper.

❼ Allow the chocolate-covered figs to harden for about 30 minutes in refrigerator and enjoy.

Calories: 97; Fat 3g; Protein 0.5g; Carb. 16g; Fiber 3.4g; Sugar 11.7g
Freebies: 0.8 FRUIT; 0.6 FAT

References

Alcohol and Weight Loss

Flechtner-Mors, M. et al. (2004). Effects of moderate consumption of white wine on weight loss in overweight and obese subjects. *International Journal of Obesity, 24,* 1420–1426.

Tolstrup, J. S. et al. (2008). Alcohol drinking frequency in relation to subsequent changes in waist circumference. *American Journal of Clinical Nutrition, 87,* 957–963.

Appetite Regulation

Ahima, R. S., & Antwi, A. A. (2008). Brain regulation of appetite and satiety. *Endocrinology & Metabolism Clinics of North America, 37,* 811–823.

Carlson, O. et al. (2007). Impact of reduced meal frequency without caloric restriction on glucose regulation in healthy, normal weight middle-aged men and women. *Metabolism, 56,* 1729–1734.

Crespo, M. A. et al. (2009). Las hormonas gastrointestinales en el control de la ingesta de alimentos. *Endocrinología y Nutrición, 56*(6), 317–30.

Farshchi, H. R., Taylor, M. A., & Macdonald, I. A. (2005). Beneficial metabolic effects of regular meal frequency on dietary thermogenesis, insulin sensitivity, and fasting lipid profiles in healthy obese women. *American Journal of Clinical Nutrition, 81,* 16–24.

Gardiner, J. V., Jayasena, C. N., & Bloom, S. R. (2008). *Journal of Neuroendocrinology, 20,* 834–841.

Hameed, S., Dhillo, W. S., & Bloom, S. R. (2008). Gut hormones and appetite control. *Oral Diseases, 15,* 18–26.

Huda, M. S. B., Wilding, J. P. J., & Pinkney, J. H. (2006). Gut peptides and the regulation of appetite. *International Association for the Study of Obesity, 7,* 163–182.

Lowe, M. R., & Butryn, M. L. (2007). Hedonic hunger: A new dimension of appetite? *Physiology & Behavior, 97,* 432–439.

Magni, P. et al. (2009). Feeding behavior in mammals including humans. *Trends in Comparative Endocrinology & Neurobiology, 1163,* 221–232.

Minor, R. K., Chang, J. W., de Cabo, R. (2009). Hungry for life: How the arcuate nucleus and neuropeptide Y may play a critical role in mediating the benefits of calorie restriction. *Molecular Cellular Endocrinology, 299*(1), 79–81.

Neary, M. T., & Batterham, R. L. (2009). Gut hormones: Implications for the treatment of obesity. *Pharmacology & Therapeutics, 124,* 44–56.

Woods, S. C., & D'Alessio, D. A. (2008). Central control of body weight and appetite. *Journal of Clinical Endocrinology & Metabolism, 93*(11), 537–550.

Wynne, K. et al. (2005). Appetite control. *Journal of Endocrinology, 184,* 291–318.

Carbohydrate and Brain Function

Dye, L., Lluch, A., & Blundell, J. E. (2000). Macronutrients and mental performance. *Nutrition, 16,* 1021–1034.

Lieberman, H. R. (2003). Nutrition, brain function and cognitive performance. *Appetite, 40*, 245–254.

Wurtman, R. J. (1986). Ways that food can affect the brain. *Nutrition Reviews, 44* (suppl.53), 2–6.

Exercise Not for Weight Loss

Achten, J., & Jeukendrup, A. E. (2004). Optimizing fat oxidation through exercise and diet. *Nutrition, 20,* 716–727.

American College of Sports Medicine. (2009). Position of the American Dietetic Association: Weight management. *Journal of the American Dietetic Association, 109*(2), 330–342.

Caudwell, P. et al. (2009). Exercise alone is not enough: Weight loss also needs a healthy (Mediterranean) diet? *Public Health Nutrition, 12*(9A), 1663–1666.

Church, T. S. et al. (2009). Changes in weight, waist circumference and compensatory responses with different doses of exercise among sedentary, overweight postmenopausal women. *PLoS ONE, 4*(2), e4515..

Finlayson, G. et al. (2009). Acute compensatory eating following exercise is associated with implicit hedonic wanting for food. *Physiology & Behavior, 97,* 62–67.

Hagobian, T. A., & Braun, B. (2010). Physical activity and hormonal regulation of appetite: Sex differences and weight control. *Exercise and Sport Sciences Reviews, 38*(1), 25–30.

Hagobian, T. A., Sharoff, C. G., & Braun B. (2008). Effects of short-term exercise and energy surplus on hormones related to regulation of energy balance. *Metabolism, 57(3),* 393–398.

Jakicic, J. M., & Otto, A. D. (2008). Physical activity considerations for the treatment and prevention of obesity. *American Journal of Clinical Nutrition, 82,* 226S–229S.

Kaushik, S. et al. (2011). Autophagy in hypothalamic AgRP neurons regulates food intake and energy balance. *Cell Metabolism, 14,* 173–183.

King et al. (2007). Metabolic and behavioral compensatory responses to exercise interventions: Barriers to weight loss. *Obesity, 15*(6), 1373–1383.

Melanson, E. L., MacLean, P. S., & Holl, J. O. (2009). Exercise improves fat metabolism in muscle but does not increase 24-h fat oxidation. *Exercise and Sports Science Reviews, 37*(2), 93–101.

Muraven, M., & Baumeister, R. F. (2000). Self-regulation and depletion of limited resources: Does self-control resemble a muscle? *Psychological Bulletin, 126*(2), 247–259.

Okay, D. M. et al. (2009). Exercise and obesity. *Primary Care: Clinics in Office Practice, 36,* 379–393.

Poirier, P., & Despres, J. P. (2001). Exercise in weight management of obesity. *Cardiology Clinics, 19*(3), 459–466.

Redman, L. M. et al. (2009). Effect of calorie restriction with or without exercise on body composition and fat distribution. *Journal of Clinical Endocrinology & Metabolism, 92*(3), 865–872.

Reynolds, G. (April 18, 2010). Weighing the evidence on exercise: Does working out really help you lose weight—or keep it off? *New York Times Magazine,* pp. 36, 41.

Sonneville, K. R., & Gortmaker, S. L. (2008). Total energy intake, adolescent discretionary behaviors and the energy gap. *International Journal of Obesity, 32,* 519–527.

Stiegler, P., & Cunliffe, A. (2006). The role of diet and exercise for the maintenance of fat-free mass and resting metabolic rate during weight loss. *Sports Medicine, 36*(3), 239–262.

Strasser, B., Spreitzer, A., Haber, P. (2007). Fat loss depends on energy deficit only, independently of the method for weight loss. *Annals of Nutrition & Metabolism, 51,* 428–432.

Swinburn, B. A. et al. (2009). Estimating the changes in energy flux that characterize the rise in obesity prevalence. *American Journal of Clinical Nutrition, 89,* 1–6.

Thacker, S. B. et al. (2004). The impact of stretching on sports injury risk: A systematic review of the literature. *Clinical Journal of Sport Medicine, 36,* 371–378.

Tremblay, A., & Buemann, B. (1995). Exercise-training, macronutrient balance and body weight control. *International Journal of Obesity, 19,* 79–86.

Volek, J. S., VanHeest, J. L., & Forsythe, C. E. (2005). Diet and exercise for weight loss. *Sports Medicine, 35*(1), 1–9.

Ghrelin and Exercise

Ballard, T. P. et al. (2009). Effect of resistance exercise, with or without carbohydrate supplementation, on plasma ghrelin concentrations and postexercise hunger and food intake. *Metabolism Clinical and Experimental, 58,* 1191–1199.

Broom, D. R. et al. (2007). Exercise-induced suppression of acylated ghrelin in humans. *American Journal of Psychology Regulatory, Integrative and Comparative Psychology, 102,* R2165–R2171.

Broom, D. R. et al. (2008). Influence of resistance and aerobic exercise on hunger, circulating levels of acylated ghrelin, and peptide YY in healthy males. *American Journal of Psychology Regulatory, Integrative and Comparative Psychology, 296,* R29–R35.

Burns, S. F. et al. (2007). A single session of treadmill running has no effect on plasma total ghrelin concentrations. *Journal of Sports Sciences, 25*(6), 635–642.

DeSouza, M. J. et al. (2004). Fasting ghrelin levels in physically active women: Relationship with menstrual disturbances and metabolic hormones. *Journal of Clinical Endocrinology & Metabolism, 89*(7), 3536–3542.

Hagobian, T. A. et al. (2008). Effects of exercise on energy-regulating hormones and appetite in men and women. *American Journal of Psychology Regulatory, Integrative and Comparative Psychology, 296,* R233–R242.

Kraemer, R. R., & Castracane, V. D. (2007). Exercise and humoral mediators of peripheral energy balance: Ghrelin and adiponectin. *Society for Experimental Biology and Medicine,* 184–191.

Leidy, H. J. et al. (2004). Circulating ghrelin is sensitive to changes in body weight during a diet and exercise program in normal young women. *Journal of Clinical*

Endocrinology & Metabolism, 89(6), 2659–2664.

Mackelvie, K. J. et al. (2007). Regulation of appetite in lean and obese adolescents after exercise: Role of acylated and desacyl ghrelin. *Journal of Clinical Endocrinology & Metabolism, 92*(2), 648–654.

Malkova, D. et al. (2008). Effect of moderate-intensity exercise session on preprandial and postprandial responses of circulating ghrelin and appetite. *Hormone and Metabolic Research, 40,* 410–415.

Martins, C. et al. (2007). Effects of exercise on gut peptides, energy increase and appetite. *Journal of Endocrinology, 193,* 251–258.

Martins, C., Morgan, L. & Truby, H. (2008). A review of the effects of exercise on appetite regulation: An obesity perspective. *International Journal of Obesity, 32,* 1337–1347.

Purell, J. Q., Cummings, D., & Weigle, D. S. (2007). Changes in 24-h area-under-the-curve ghrelin values following diet-induced weight loss are associated with loss of fat-free mass, but not with changes in fat mass, insulin levels or insulin sensitivity. *International Journal of Obesity, 31,* 385–389.

St.-Pierre, D. H. et al. (2004). Relationship between ghrelin and energy expenditure in healthy young women. *Journal of Clinical Endocrinology & Metabolism, 89*(12), 5993–5997.

Ghrelin and Food

Blom, W. A. M. et al. (2005). Ghrelin response to carbohydrate-enriched breakfast is related to insulin. *American Journal of Clinical Nutrition, 81,* 367–375.

Crujeriras, A. B. et al. (2010). Weight regain after a diet-induced loss is predicted by higher baseline leptin and lower ghrelin plasma levels. *Journal of Clinical Endocrinology Metabolism, 95*(1), 5037–5044.

Cummings, D. E. (2006). Ghrelin and the short- and long-term regulation of appetite and body weight. *Physiology & Behavior, 89,* 71–84.

Cummings, D. E. et al. (2001). A preprandial rise in plasma ghrelin levels suggests a role in meal initiation in humans. *Diabetes, 50,* 1714–1719.

Cummings, D. E. et al. (2004). Plasma ghrelin levels and hunger scores in humans initiating meals voluntarily without time- and food-related cues. *American Journal of Physiology—Endocrinology & Metabolism, 287,* E297–E304.

Depoortere, I. (2009). Targeting the ghrelin receptor to regulate food intake. *Regulatory Peptides, 156,* 13–23.

DeVriese, C., & Delporte, C. (2007). Influence of ghrelin on food intake and energy homeostasis. *Current Opinion in Clinical Nutrition and Metabolic Care, 10,* 615–619.

Erdmann, J. et al. (2004). Postprandial response of plasma ghrelin levels to various test meals in relation to food intake, plasma insulin, and glucose. *Journal of Endocrinology & Metabolism, 89*(6), 3048–3054.

Foster-Schubert, K. E. et al. (2008). Acyl and total ghrelin are suppressed strongly by ingested proteins, weakly by lipids, and biphasically by carbohydrates. *Journal of Clinical Endocrinology & Metabolism, 93*(5), 1971–1979.

Kola, B., & Korbonits, M. (2009). Shedding light on the intricate puzzle of ghrelin's effects on appetite regulation. *Journal of Endocrinology, 202,* 191–198.

Leidy, H. J., Mattes, R. D., & Campbell, W. W. (2007). Effects of acute and chronic protein intake on metabolism, appetite, and ghrelin during weight loss. *Obesity, 15*(2), 1215–1225.

Leidy, H. J., & Williams, N. I. (2006). Meal energy content is related to features of meal-related ghrelin profiles across a typical day of eating in non-obese premenopausal women. *Hormone and Metabolic Research, 38,* 317–322.

Levin, F. et al. (2006). Ghrelin stimulates gastric emptying and hunger in normal-weight humans. *Journal of Endocrinology & Metabolism, 91*(9), 3296–3302.

Natalucci, G. et al. (2005). Spontaneous 24-h ghrelin secretion pattern in fasting subjects: Maintenance of a meal-related pattern. *European Journal of Endocrinology, 152,* 845–850.

Pusztai, P. et al. (2008). Ghrelin: A new peptide regulating the neurohormonal system, energy homeostasis and glucose metabolism. *Diabetes Metabolism Research and Reviews, 24,* 343–352.

St.-Pierre, D. H. et al. (2006). Lifestyle behaviours and components of energy balance as independent predictors of ghrelin and adiponectin in young non-obese women. *Diabetes Metabolism, 32,* 131–139.

Wren A. M., et al. (2009). Ghrelin enhances appetite and increases food intake in humans. *Journal of Clinical Endocrinology & Metabolism, 86,* 5992–5995.

Yin, X. et al. (2009). Ghrelin fluctuation, what determines its production? *Acta Biochemica Biophysica Sinica, 41*(3), 188–197.

Global Obesity

Berghofer, A. et al. (2008). Obesity prevalence from a European perspective: A systematic review. *BioMed Central Public Health, 8,* 200.

Charles, M. A., Eschwege, E., & Basdevant, A. (2008). Monitoring the obesity epidemic in France: The Obepi surveys, 1997–2006. *Obesity, 16*(9), 2182–2186.

Chen, C. M. (2008). Overview of obesity in mainland China. *International Association for the Study of Obesity, 9*(1), 14–21.

Gallus, S. et al. (2006). Overweight and obesity in Italian adults 2004, and an overview of trends since 1983. *European Journal of Clinical Nutrition, 60,* 1174–1179.

Gill, T. (2006). Epidemiology and health impact of obesity: An Asia Pacific perspective. *Asia Pacific Journal of Clinical Nutrition, 15,* 3–14.

Micciolo, R. et al. (2010). Prevalence of overweight and obesity in Italy (2001–2001): Is there a rising obesity epidemic? *AEP, 20*(4), 258–264.

Pigeyre, M. et al. (2011). Effects of occupational and educational changes on obesity trends in France: The results of the MONICA-France survey, 1986–2006. *Preventive Medicine, 52,* 305–309.

Rozin, P. et al. (2003). The ecology of eating: Smaller portion sizes in France than in the United States help explain the French paradox. *Psychological Science, 14*(5), 450–454.

Sanchez, J., et al. (2006). *Encuesta Nacional de Indicadores Nutricionales, Bioquímicos, Socioeconomicos y Culturales Relacionados con las Enfermedades Crónicas Degenerativas.* Lima, Peru: Ministerio de Salud.

Wang, Y. et al. (2007). Is China facing an obesity epidemic and the consequences? The trends in obesity and chronic disease in China. *International Journal of Obesity, 31,* 177–188.

Meal Frequency

Farshchi, H. R., Taylor, M. A., & Macdonald, I. A. (2004). Regular meal frequency creates more appropriate insulin sensitivity and lipid profiles compared with irregular meal frequency in healthy lean women. *European Journal of Clinical Nutrition, 58,* 1071–1077.

Sleep Cycles

Coe, S. (2011). Can a poor night's sleep stop you from losing body fat? *Nutrition Bulletin, 36,* 99–101.

Hairston, K. G. et al. (2010). Sleep duration and five-year abdominal fat accumulation in a minority cohort: The IRAS family study. *Sleep, 33*(3), 289–295.

Stress and Eating/Health

Anderson, D. A. et al. (2002). Self-reported dietary restraint is associated with elevated levels of salivary cortisol. *Appetite, 38,* 13–17.

Block, J. P. et al. (2009). Psychosocial stress and change in weight among US adults. *American Journal of Epidemiology, 170,* 181–192.

Cameron, M. J., Maguire, R. W., McCormack, J. (2001). Stress-induced binge eating: A behavior analytic approach to assessment and intervention. *Journal of Adult Development 18,* 81–84.

George, S. A. et al. (2010). CRH-stimulated cortisol release and food intake in healthy, non-obese adults. *Psychoneuroendocrinology, 35,* 607–612.

Kandiah, J., Yake, M., Willett, H. (2008). Effects of stress on eating practices among adults. *Family & Consumer Sciences Research Journal, 37*(1), 27–38.

Martens. M. J. I. et al. (2010). Effects of single macronutrients on serum cortisol concentrations in normal weight men. *Physiology & Behavior, 101,* 563–567.

Tomiyama, J. et al. (2010). Low calorie dieting increases cortisol. *Psychosomatic Medicine, 72*(4), 357–364.

Torres, S. J., & Nowson, C. A. (2007). Relationship between stress, eating behavior, and obesity. *Nutrition, 23,* 887–894.

Vicennati, V. et al. (2011). Cortisol, energy intake, and food frequency in overweight/obese women. *Nutrition, 27,* 677–680.

Other

Boldec, L. (2009). Are sleep disorders influencing patient's weight? *Weight Management Matters, 7*(2), 10–11.

Chaput, J. P., & Tremblay, A. (2009). The glucostatic theory of appetite control and the risk of obesity and diabetes. *International Journal of Obesity, 33*, 46–53.

Dye, L., & Blundell, J. E. (1997). Menstrual cycle and appetite control: Implications for weight regulation. *Human Reproduction, 12*(6), 1142–1151.

Eckel, R. H. (2008). Obesity research in the next decade. *International Journal of Obesity, 32*, S143–S151.

Flegal , K. H., Carroll, M. D., Ogden, C. L., & Johnson, C. L. (2002). Prevalence and trends in obesity among US adults, 1999–2000. *Journal of American Medical Association, 288* (14), 1723–1727.

Johnstone, A. M. (2007). Fasting—the ultimate diet? *Obesity Reviews, 8*, 211–222.

Sacks, F. M. et al. (2009). Comparison of weight-loss diets with different compositions of fat, protein, and carbohydrates. *New England Journal of Medicine, 360*(9), 859–873.

Appendix A

Average Total Energy Expenditure

	MALES				FEMALES		
ACTIVITY LEVEL	Sedentary	Moderate Active	Active	ACTIVITY LEVEL	Sedentary	Moderate Active	Active
AGE				AGE			
18	2400	2800	3200	18	1800	2000	2400
19–20	2600	2800	3000	19–20	2000	2200	2400
21–25	2400	2800	3000	21–25	2000	2200	2400
26–30	2400	2600	3000	26–30	1800	2000	2400
31–35	2400	2600	3000	31–35	1800	2000	2200
36–40	2400	2600	2800	36–40	1800	2000	2200
41–45	2200	2600	2800	41–45	1800	2000	2200
46–50	2200	2400	2800	46–50	1800	2000	2200
51–55	2200	2400	2800	51–55	1600	1800	2200
56–60	2200	2400	2600	56–60	1600	1800	2200
61–65	2000	2400	2600	61–65	1600	1800	2000
66–70	2000	2200	2600	66–70	1600	1800	2000
71–75	2000	2200	2600	71–75	1600	1800	2000

Calorie levels are based on the Estimated Energy Requirements and activity levels from the Institute of Medicine Dietary Reference Intakes Macronutrients Report, 2002.

Sedentary = less than 30 minutes a day of moderate physical activity in addition to daily activities.

Moderate active = at least 30 minutes up to 60 minutes a day of moderate physical activity in addition to daily activities.

Active = 60 or more minutes a day of moderate physical activity in addition to daily activities.

Source: *USDA Dietary Guidelines for Americans: 2005*

Appendix B

Shopping list for the 7-day sample menus

Grains & Starches

Breads:

Select the bread of your choice or the ones used below in the seven-day sample menus.

- ❏ Bread, Whole Grain, Rice or Corn *(3g or more fiber, 80–100 kcal/slice)*
- ❏ Dark Rye Bread
- ❏ English Muffins, Whole Grain
- ❏ Pita Pocket Bread, Whole Grain

Cereals:

Choose cereals that have 5g or more of fiber and 6g or less of sugar per serving

Crackers/Crisps

Choose crackers/crisps that have 4g or more of fiber and 2g or less of fat per serving.

Grains:

- ❏ Pasta, Whole Grain, Rice or Quinoa
- ❏ Rice, Brown or Jasmine
- ❏ Quinoa
- ❏ Beans *(any kind, canned or dried)*
- ❏ Oatmeal *(flakes or steel cut)* or Gluten-Free Oats

Starchy Vegetables:

- ❏ Sweet Potatoes

Tortillas:

- ❏ Corn tortilla, 5" in diameter

Milk, Dairy and Dairy Alternatives

Milk:

- ❏ Fat-Free Milk or Low-Fat *(1%)* Milk

Yogurt:

- ❏ Greek Yogurt, fat free

Milk Alternative:

- ❏ Soy, Rice or Almond Milk, 3g or less of fat per serving

Creams:

- ❏ Whipped Light Cream

Meats and Vegetarian Meats:

4% or less fat (2g or less of fat per ounce in weight):

❑ Chicken *(white meat only, no skin)*

❑ Deli Cold Cuts: Turkey, Ham *(nitrites free)*

❑ Tuna *(white fish, canned, packed in water)* or Salmon *(fresh, frozen, or canned in water)*

❑ Smoked Salmon

❑ Shrimp *(fresh or frozen)*

❑ Ground Turkey

❑ Fish Fillets *(fresh or frozen)*

❑ Eggs

❑ Cottage Cheese, fat-free or low-fat 1%

7% or less fat (3g or less of fat per ounce in weight):

❑ Grated Parmesan Cheese

❑ Cheddar Cheese, low-fat

❑ Spreadable Cheese, low-fat

❑ Cheese Snack Sticks, Mozzarella or Mild Cheddar, low-fat

10% or less fat (5g or less of fat per ounce in weight):

❑ Chicken Sausage

❑ Fruits

❑ Eat fruits from every color group each and every week. Try to buy seasonal and locally grown produce and support our farmers' markets, or frozen fruits are a good alternative.

Here are fruits that are used in the 7-day sample menus:

❑ Blueberries, Figs

❑ Cantaloupe, Mango, Apricots, Pineapple

❑ Strawberries, Watermelon, Apple-

❑ Lemon, Lime

Vegetables:

❑ Eat vegetables from every color group each and every week. Try to buy seasonal and locally grown produce and support our farmers' markets, and frozen vegetables are a good alternative.

Here are vegetables that are used in the 7-day sample menus:

❑ Tomato or Vegetable Soup

❑ Tomatoes, Red Onions, Shallots

❑ Carrots, Bell Peppers

❑ Celery, Asparagus, Romaine Lettuce, Spinach, Salad Mix, Argula, Green Beans, Cucumbers, Snap Peas, Broccoli

Fats:

- ❏ Almonds or Walnuts
- ❏ Avocado
- ❏ Olive Oil
- ❏ Butter
- ❏ Ground Flaxseed
- ❏ Shredded Coconut, sweetened

Desserts:

- ❏ Light Vanilla Ice Cream
- ❏ Dark Chocolate, 70% or more dark

Sauces and Condiments:

- ❏ Choose a tomato sauce that has 1g or less of fat and 3g or less of sugar per ½ cup serving
- ❏ Capers
- ❏ Cream Cheese, Low-Fat or Fat-Free
- ❏ Dijon Mustard
- ❏ Extra Strong Instant Coffee
- ❏ Maple Syrup
- ❏ Paprika
- ❏ Salad Dressing, Low-Fat or Fat-Free
- ❏ Salsa
- ❏ Vinegar *(red or white wine, malt, or apple cider)*
- ❏ Optional: dried red chili flakes, salt, pepper

Note: This shopping list reflects the seven-day sample menus. However, it does not include the ingredients needed in the individual recipes within the sample menus. Please refer to the recipe list for ingredients needed.

Index

About the Author

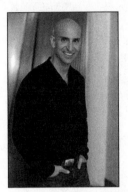

Manuel Villacorta is a registered dietitian and certified specialist in sports dietetics with more than 16 years of experience. He is one of the leading weight loss and nutrition experts in the United States, acting as a national media spokesperson for the Academy of Nutrition and Dietetics, a health blog contributor for *The Huffington Post*, an on-air contributor for the Univision television network, and a health and lifestyle contributor for Fox News Latino. Manuel is the owner of San Francisco–based private practice, MV Nutrition, and the recipient of three consecutive "Best Bay Area Nutritionist" awards (2008, 2009, and 2010) from the *San Francisco Chronicle* and Citysearch.

His warm, approachable style and his bilingual proficiency in English and Spanish have made him an in-demand health and nutrition expert on local and national television and radio channels, as well as in articles appearing in print publications and online.

Manuel is a compelling, charismatic communicator. As a speaker, he is often praised for making audiences feel heard, motivated, and engaged. He is often invited to speak at annual state and national conventions for organizations, associations, and corporations as part of their wellness strategy. Known to educate team members about the truth surrounding food, Manuel empowers his audiences to make the right choices and motivates them to take charge on their own health. According to many clients, Manuel's enthusiasm and encouragement has changed their lives.

Manuel earned his bachelor of science in nutrition and physiology metabolism from the University of California, Berkeley, and his master of science in nutrition and food science from San Jose State University. He has been the recipient of numerous prestigious awards for his research and contributions to the field of dietetics.

Look What *Eating Free* Did for These People . . .

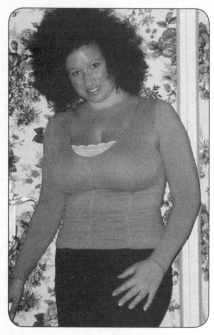

Denise: Before

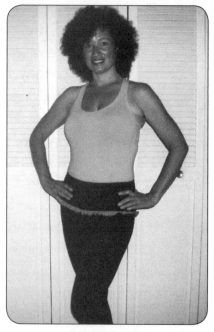

Denise: After

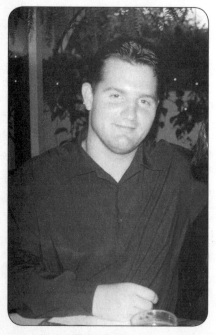

Eric: Before

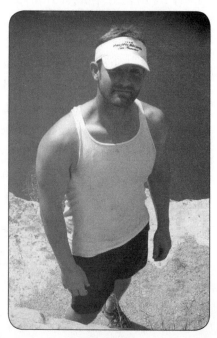

Eric: After

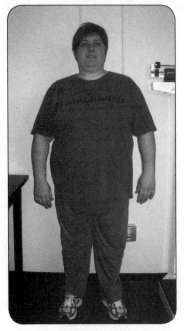

Kelley: Before

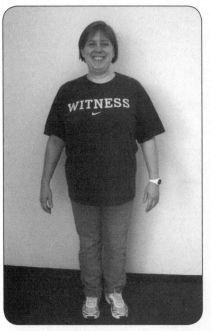

Kelley: After

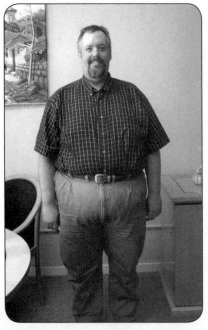

Kevin: Before

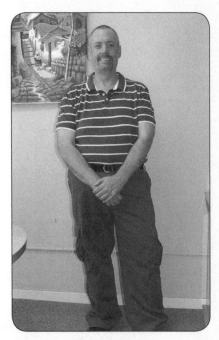

Kevin: After

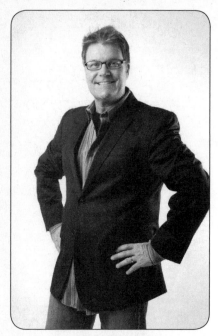

Paul: Before

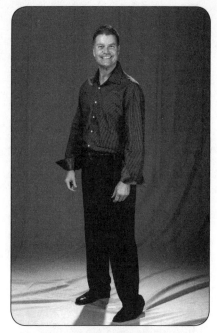

Paul: After

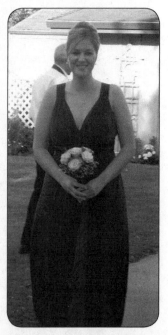

Samantha: Before

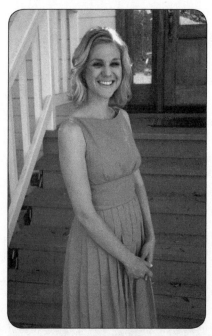

Samantha: After